ABSOLUTE BEGINNER'S GUIDE

TO

Half-Marathon Training

Heather Hedrick, M.S., R.D.

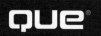

800 East 96th Street,
Indianapolis, Indiana 46240

Absolute Beginner's Guide to Half-Marathon Training

International Standard Book Number: 0-7897-3314-5

Library of Congress Catalog Card Number: 2004114914

Printed in the United States of America

First Printing: December 2004
Reprinted with corrections: October 2008

10 11 12   11 10 9 8

Trademarks

All terms mentioned in this book that are known to be trademarks or service marks have been appropriately capitalized. Que Publishing cannot attest to the accuracy of this information. Use of a term in this book should not be regarded as affecting the validity of any trademark or service mark.

Warning and Disclaimer

Every effort has been made to make this book as complete and as accurate as possible, but no warranty or fitness is implied. The information provided is on an "as is" basis. The author and the publisher shall have neither liability nor responsibility to any person or entity with respect to any loss or damages arising from the information contained in this.

Bulk Sales

Que Publishing offers excellent discounts on this book when ordered in quantity for bulk purchases or special sales. For more information, please contact

U.S. Corporate and Government Sales
1-800-382-3419
corpsales@pearsontechgroup.com

For sales outside of the U.S., please contact

International Sales
international@pearsoned.com

Executive Editor
Candace Hall

Acquisitions Editor
Karen Whitehouse

Development Editor
Sean Dixon

Managing Editor
Charlotte Clapp

Project Editor
Andy Beaster

Copy Editor
Kate Givens

Indexer
Chris Barrick

Publishing Coordinator
Cindy Teeters

Interior Designer
Anne Jones

Cover Designer
Dan Armstrong

Page Layout
Julie Parks

Contents at a Glance

Table of Contents

About the Author

Heather Hedrick is the assistant director of the Center for Educational Services within the National Institute for Fitness and Sport. She is a registered dietitian and has her Master of Science in Kinesiology. She completed her Bachelor of Science degree in dietetics as well as her Master of Science degree at the University of Illinois, Urbana/Champaign. Heather is certified by the American College of Sports Medicine as a Health/Fitness Instructor®. Heather's interests and extensive experience are in the areas of wellness, weight management, exercise programming, vegetarian nutrition, and sports nutrition, ranging from the recreational to the ultra-endurance athlete. At the National Institute for Fitness and Sport, she develops educational materials, implements programs, and delivers presentations to various groups on nutrition and fitness topics related to healthy eating, weight control, disease prevention, and improving athletic performance. Heather coordinates the National Institute for Fitness and Sport's Mini Marathon Training Program—a half-marathon training program for walkers and runners participating in the 500 Festival Mini Marathon, the nation's largest half-marathon. She routinely appears on local NBC, CBS, and cable television shows and news broadcasts to educate central Indiana residents on the benefits of a healthy lifestyle. She was the dietitian for the first team of four men aged 70+ to successfully complete the non-stop bicycle race, Race Across America. Heather has authored nutrition/fitness articles published in a variety of journals including *Mechanisms of Ageing and Development* and the *ACSM Health & Fitness® Journal*. She has been interviewed and quoted in *Women's Day, Ladies Home Journal*, and *Newsweek* magazines. Heather is also an accomplished triathlete, duathlete, and marathon runner, including qualifying and competing in the 2003 Hawaii Ironman.

Dedication

To my parents, Brad and Carol Hedrick, who taught me that with hard work and dedication, anything is possible.

Acknowledgments

I would like to acknowledge the hard work and dedication of the past and current National Institute for Fitness and Sport interns, as well as my colleagues who have contributed their knowledge and expertise on training for 5Ks, 10Ks, and half-marathons. My co-worker and friend, Nicole Haywood, deserves special recognition for her daily support and good humor. Thank you to my running and triathlon training partners who have kept me company while I practice what I preach. My greatest appreciation is for my family and friends whose love and encouragement keep me motivated and inspired.

We Want to Hear from You!

As the reader of this book, *you* are our most important critic and commentator. We value your opinion and want to know what we're doing right, what we could do better, what areas you'd like to see us publish in, and any other words of wisdom you're willing to pass our way.

As an executive editor for Que Publishing, I welcome your comments. You can email or write me directly to let me know what you did or didn't like about this book—as well as what we can do to make our books better.

Please note that I cannot help you with technical problems related to the topic of this book. We do have a User Services group, however, where I will forward specific technical questions related to the book.

When you write, please be sure to include this book's title and author as well as your name, email address, and phone number. I will carefully review your comments and share them with the author and editors who worked on the book.

Email: feedback@quepublishing.com

Mail: Candace Hall
Executive Editor
Que Publishing
800 East 96th Street
Indianapolis, IN 46240 USA

For more information about this book or another Que title, visit our website at www.quepublishing.com. Type the ISBN (excluding hyphens) or the title of a book in the Search field to find the page you're looking for.

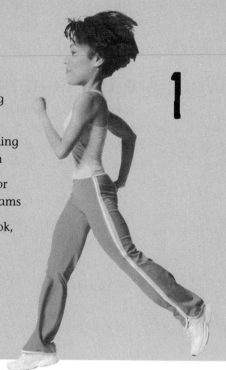

IN THIS CHAPTER

- Physical and mental benefits of walking and running

- Profile of an individual capable of walking or running a 5K, 10K, or half-marathon

- Background on the National Institute for Fitness and Sport and its training programs

- Overview of the key concepts of this book, including unique features

1

INTRODUCTION

You can do it!

Many people view the successful completion of a 5K, 10K, or half-marathon as impossible. However, if you possess the desire and the dedication, you *can* do it. Making the commitment to train for an endurance event such as a 5K, 10K, or half-marathon is one that you will not regret. So lace up your shoes, get fired up, and let the training begin!

What Are the Benefits of Walking and Running?

Congratulations for exploring the world of walking and running! Exercising on a regular basis is one of the best habits you can acquire. Over the years, physical activity research has discovered the numerous positive affects of exercise on our physical and mental health. Daily physical activity and regular exercise can reduce the risk of:

- Premature mortality
- Coronary heart disease
- Hypertension
- Certain cancers
- Osteoporosis
- Diabetes
- Obesity

Daily physical activity and regular exercise can also improve:

- Immune function
- Cholesterol levels
- Cardiovascular function
- Respiratory function
- Glucose tolerance
- Self-esteem
- Mood

The research has been so profound that in 1996 the Surgeon General published the following warning to all Americans: "The Surgeon General has determined that lack of physical activity is detrimental to your health." This was a landmark statement because it was the first time that a warning had been issued about Americans *not* doing something versus pleading with individuals to stop doing something (such as to stop smoking). The resulting recommendation was that "All Americans should acquire 30 minutes or more of moderate-intensity physical activity on most, preferably all, days of the week." By making the commitment to train for a 5K, 10K, or half-marathon, and by following the protocols presented in this book, you will be accomplishing the recommendation of exercising on most days of the week.

A well-rounded exercise program includes a balance of three components of physical fitness: cardiorespiratory fitness, muscular fitness, and flexibility. Running and walking are considered cardiorespiratory exercises. In this book, you will find information on creating a strength-training program to improve your muscular fitness, as well as guidelines for stretching to increase your flexibility. I encourage you to incorporate all three components of fitness into your weekly routine.

Who Can Train and Successfully Complete a 5K, 10K, or Half-Marathon?

Nearly anyone who has the desire and the dedication can successfully train for and complete a 5K, 10K, or half-marathon. However, there are a few exceptions. First, the protocols presented in this book are designed for individuals over the age of 16 and therefore may not meet the needs of young runners and walkers. Secondly, if you have any acute musculoskeletal injuries, have had recent surgery, or have uncontrolled chronic diseases, you should consult with your physician before embarking on a walking or running program. Finally, if you have never been physically active, I suggest you make an appointment with your physician to discuss any appropriate modifications to your 5K, 10K, or half-marathon training based on your past and current medical history.

Why Should You Follow the National Institute for Fitness and Sport's (NIFS) Training Programs?

There are many different types of training programs available in books, online, and from private coaches. With so many options available, why should you follow the guidelines in this book? The answer can be summed up with three words: education, experience, and success. The mission of NIFS is centered on the health, fitness, and well being of individuals of all ages and abilities. The driving force behind this book is to educate and empower individuals to accomplish their physical activity goals through walking and running. NIFS staff is university-degreed and certified by national organizations in the areas of fitness, nutrition, and health. In addition to a formal education, the NIFS staff is also composed of accomplished athletes who practice what they preach. The NIFS running and walking training programs have helped thousands of people successfully accomplish their long-distance walking and running goals. With the combination of education, experience, and success, all you need is the desire and dedication; this book will give you the tools to accomplish your 5K, 10K, and half-marathon goals.

How Did NIFS Originate?

NIFS is a not-for-profit organization located on the Indiana University-Purdue University at Indianapolis (IUPUI) campus in downtown Indianapolis, Indiana. The concept for NIFS began in June 1983, when the President's Council on Physical Fitness and Sport announced that Indianapolis was selected as the site for a U.S. Fitness Academy. In 1984, the Academy staff decided to pursue development in California—but community leaders in Indianapolis pledged to carry forth with plans for a major center for health and physical fitness research, education, and service in the city. In 1985, funding pledges from Lilly Endowment, Inc., the State of Indiana, and the City of Indianapolis made the dream possible. Groundbreaking took place on May 9, 1985, and the first board meeting and cornerstone ceremony took place September 11, 1986. In June 1988, the staff moved from temporary quarters in the IUPUI Natatorium building to the new facility at 250 University Boulevard, Indianapolis, IN.

November 1, 1988, marked the dedication of the facility and the opening of the Fitness Center, which now has more than 4,000 members. Since 1988, the NIFS staff has conducted more than 5,000 graded exercise tests for Indiana state police troopers, professional and amateur athletes, corporate clients, and individual members. More than 100,000 Indianapolis-area youth have benefited from NIFS field trips, athletic development programs, and youth camps. Service, research, and educational programs have reached thousands more.

NIFS fitness, wellness, and athletic programs are designed to benefit all, from the ranks of the professional and amateur athlete to the fitness enthusiast to children and adults of all ages and abilities.

note

NIFS Mission Statement: The National Institute for Fitness and Sport is committed to enhancing human health, physical fitness, and athletic performance through research, education, and service.

How Does NIFS Accomplish Its Mission?

The mission of NIFS is carried out through six centers, each working together as an integrated team. The six centers include:

- *Indiana University Medical Group at NIFS*—This center offers medical consultation and services in the areas of asthma, allergies, pulmonary medicine, neurosurgery, pediatric orthopeadic surgery, as well as a comprehensive executive physical program.
- *Fitness Center*—The Fitness Center is a 66,000 square foot, state-of-the-art training facility, serving people of all ages and abilities. A highly trained and

qualified staff works one-on-one with members to develop exercise prescriptions and specialized training programs based on individual fitness assessments.

- *Athletic Development*—This center designs rigorous training programs that maximize the athletic skills of both children and adults. The Athletic Development services are designed to help all athletes (regardless of sport, age, or ability) to improve skills such as explosive power, coordination, speed, strength, agility, and mental toughness.

- *Educational Services*—Educational Services works in conjunction with all the NIFS centers to provide health/fitness, nutrition, and wellness services and programs to corporate clients, community clients, and professionals. Services include training workshops, wellness and health education presentations, nutrition consultations, weight management programs, corporate team building, and a large-scale half-marathon training program.

- *Corporate Fitness Management*—Corporate Fitness Management specializes in the day-to-day operations of NIFS off-site corporate fitness facilities and the development, implementation, promotion, and evaluation of worksite health and wellness programs. Included are membership, marketing/promotion, health screenings, fitness testing, exercise prescription, personal training, health and wellness education, and motivation/incentive programs.

- *Youth Development*—This center offers fun, high-quality programs and field trips for children ages 3–17 that are success-oriented, non-competitive, and non-sport specific. The philosophy in the Center for Youth Development is "learning to move and learning through movement."

What Is the NIFS Mini Marathon Training Program?

NIFS conducts an annual half-marathon training program for walkers and runners in central Indiana. The NIFS program, in its 15th year, has been developed by exercise physiologists, fitness specialists, and registered dietitians to help participants maximize their safety, performance, and enjoyment of training for a half-marathon. The program runs January through May to help locals prepare for the 500 Festival Mini Marathon, which is the largest half-marathon in the nation. Five hundred to six hundred people join the NIFS half-marathon training program every year. Participants successfully complete the 13.1 mile journey from downtown Indianapolis to the track at the Indianapolis Motor Speedway (the location of the Indianapolis 500) and back downtown.

With the educational background of the NIFS staff, the knowledge and experience of how to empower people to achieve their health and fitness goals, and the successful history of helping walkers and runners train for and complete 5Ks, 10Ks, and half-marathons, you are in good hands!

PAST PARTICIPANTS SPEAK UP

"I wanted to thank you for all your help and encouragement…I cut 10 minutes off my time from last year and I know I couldn't have done it without your help!"–Tim

"My experience can be summed up in one word—Professionalism, with a capital P. From the staff leaders to the volunteers, and your state-of-the-art facility at NIFS. Thanks for your great program!"–Brian

"We have participated in other training programs in the past and in my opinion the NIFS program beats theirs hands down."–Jennifer

"This was the first time I completed training for a half-marathon injury-free and the first time I reached my goal to break two hours hours for the race. It's great to be reaching my 40th birthday having done something physical I couldn't do at my 30th."–Eric

---

What Are the Unique Features of This Book?

The information in this book will provide all the tools you need to accomplish your 5K, 10K, and half-marathon goals. You will begin by setting specific goals and learning how to track your progress to keep you moving in the right direction. You will learn how to calculate your target heart rate ranges and how to use the RPE scale because monitoring your exercise intensity is critical for your health, safety, and comfort.

Several chapters discuss exercising safely to prevent injuries and provide practical advice on equipment, apparel, training procedures, and running and walking form. To encourage you to create balance in your weekly routine, a chapter has been dedicated to flexibility and stretching exercises, while another chapter focuses on muscular fitness and strength training. Proper nutrition is critical for providing the fuel your body needs to successfully complete three to five days of exercise each week. Information on daily nutrition will focus on achieving balance, variety, and moderation in all of your meals and snacks; the chapter on training nutrition provides the guidelines to keep you fueled and hydrated while you are walking and running.

The last segment of this book reviews tips on how to mentally stay focused and motivated, especially on race day. My goal in providing you a well-balanced approach to training for a 5K, 10K, or half-marathon is that you will not only have fun, feel good, and successfully complete your goal, but also that you will get hooked on physical activity and exercise for a lifetime.

There are several other unique features of this book that will assist you in your 5K, 10K, or half-marathon training:

- *Before Heading Out the Door*—These tips provide a reminder of how to plan ahead to make your walks or runs more enjoyable, effective, and productive.

- *Running and Walking Training Gadgets*—With a plethora of equipment and apparel marketed to runners and walkers, the Running and Walking Training Gadgets will highlight the essentials that will make training more comfortable, safe, and fun.

- *Tear-out exercise and nutrition logs*—In the appendix, you will find weekly training logs, weekly nutrition logs, and strength training logs to record all of your workouts, meals, and snacks. If you go to http://www.quepublishing.com and type this book's ISBN (0789733145) into the Search field to go to this book's web page, you will find printable PDF versions of all three of these logs available for download. Recording your progress will keep you on track and can be very motivating.

THE ABSOLUTE MINIMUM

- Regular physical activity and exercise can improve your health and reduce your risk of many degenerative diseases.

- With the desire and the dedication, you *can* successfully complete a 5K, 10K, or half-marathon. However, if you have had any recent medical injuries or procedures, have uncontrolled chronic diseases, or have never been physically active, please see your physician before engaging in any form of exercise.

- The staff of the National Institute for Fitness and Sport has the education, experience, and history of success to help you not only meet your goals, but also to feel good and have fun.

- Incorporate strength training and stretching exercises into your weekly routine in addition to your walking and running.

- Enjoy yourself and get fired up!

2

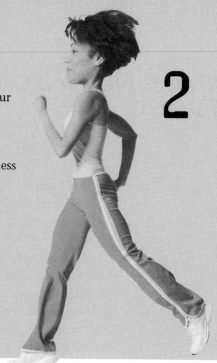

GETTING STARTED

Prepare for the adventure before embarking on the journey.

Congratulations on making the commitment to train and complete a 5K, 10K, or half-marathon! You must be eager to put on your walking or running shoes and hit the road. However, I urge you to consider a couple of things before tying up your laces. As with any endeavor, a little planning and preparation goes a long way. To prepare for 5K, 10K, and half-marathon training, you should visit your doctor for medical clearance to begin exercising or long distance training. A fitness assessment is another preparation tool that gives you information and awareness about your current fitness level, which you can use to establish fitness goals. The goal-setting process helps you to plan: Why are you training for a 5K, 10K, or half-marathon? What do you want to accomplish? What are your anticipated outcomes? By setting goals, and then tracking your progress toward those goals, you will stay on track, maintain your motivation, and ultimately be successful.

What Should You Consider Before Starting Your Training?

The 5K, 10K, and half-marathon training schedules presented in this book have been carefully designed to accommodate first-time exercisers as well as first-time long distance runners and walkers. The training schedules have been designed to increase fitness for those needing a boost or to challenge individuals to go further than they have ever gone before. While your enthusiasm and your eagerness to begin training may be piqued, there are a few things you should consider before going out for your first run or walk:

- *Check with your physician.* It is recommended that you consult with your doctor before beginning an exercise program. The American College of Sports Medicine recommends that males 45 and over, females 55 and over, or anyone with two or more major risk factors undergo a physician-supervised graded exercise test before starting a vigorous exercise program. (Major risk factors include family history of cardiovascular disease, current smoker, high blood pressure, high cholesterol, impaired fasting glucose, obesity, or sedentary lifestyle.) This is a precautionary measure to ensure you have a clean bill of health before challenging your body with physical activity.

> **note**
>
> A "sedentary lifestyle" (less than 20–30 minutes of physical activity daily) is considered a major risk factor for cardiovascular disease or complications. If you are a first-time exerciser, make sure you see your doctor before beginning your training.

- *Consider scheduling a fitness assessment.* Whether you are a first time exerciser or a regular exerciser who has not recently engaged in any walking or running, consider scheduling a fitness assessment with a certified fitness specialist. The results of the assessment will provide valuable information on your current fitness level and provide incentive for you to improve over the course of the training program. A typical fitness assessment will evaluate your cardiovascular endurance, muscular endurance, strength, flexibility, and body composition. Your areas of weakness should become a focus for your fitness goal setting.

- *Goal setting and tracking progress.* Before you begin your training, take time to consider why you want to train for a 5K, 10K, or half-marathon as well as what you hope to achieve throughout the program. The following section will detail the importance of goal setting and how to establish appropriate fitness goals. To determine your progress toward your goals, you should keep records of your daily nutrition and fitness routine throughout your training. Tracking your progress will be covered in the last section of this chapter.

Keep in mind that training for a 5K, 10K, or half-marathon is *fun*. Walking and running should be your hobby, not your job. Enjoy the process and enjoy your success.

What Is the Importance of Setting Goals?

One of the main reasons individuals drop out of an exercise program is due to lack of motivation. Everyone is internally motivated in a different way; however, setting goals is universally recognized as a key to success in sticking with an exercise plan. Goals create a vision of future accomplishments and provide the "dangling carrot" to keep you moving in the right direction.

When setting your goals, stay focused on what you want to accomplish and achieve, and avoid comparing your goals to somebody else's goals or performances. Enjoy your performance and success based on the goals you have set for yourself. Spotlighting your own accomplishments reduces stress and anxiety in trying to achieve your long-term goals.

When setting your goals, make them S.M.A.R.T. goals: **S**pecific and clearly defined; **M**easurable; **A**ttainable but challenging; **R**eward yourself; **T**ime-based.

caution

Do *not* compare your goals or performances to others. Comparisons can lead to frustration and disappointment, whereas self-focused goals can contribute to success and a great feeling of accomplishment.

Specific and Clearly Defined Goals

Identify your intentions by specifically stating how you will accomplish your goal. Vague goals often lead to half-hearted efforts, procrastination, and fewer results. Start by setting small, specific goals that will help guide you to attain your ultimate long-term goals.

Example

Nonspecific: "I will start exercising."

Specific: "I will start exercising three times a week in my training for the half-marathon."

Measurable Goals

All goals should be stated in a fashion that can be measured. By adding a value to your goals, you can more accurately determine whether you met or surpassed your expectations. Fitness goals can be measured in time, distance, heart rate, repetitions, weight, and so on; nutrition goals can be measured in portion sizes, servings per food group, ounces of fluid consumed, and so on.

Example

Nonmeasurable: "I will walk a fast 10K."

Measurable: "I will finish the 10K in 1 hour and 30 minutes."

Attainable but Challenging Goals

Set goals that will be challenging but realistic. Goals that are out of reach can be discouraging rather than motivating. Goals that are too lofty can also lead to injury. Plan to reach your goals one step at a time by setting both small, short-term goals as well as large, long-term goals.

Example

Unattainable: "I am currently training at a 9 minute/mile pace; my goal is to run the 5K at a 6 minute/mile pace."

Attainable: "I am currently training at a 9 minute/mile pace; my goal is to run the 5K at an 8:30 minute/mile pace."

Reward Yourself

Rewards are great motivators. Give yourself a prize each time you reach a goal. Reward yourself with healthy options such as new walking/running shoes, new active apparel, a massage, and so on. Do not use food as your reward as it can lead to unhealthy behaviors and relationships with food.

Example

Inappropriate Rewards: Food, desserts, or alcoholic beverages.

Appropriate Rewards: New shoes, massages, clothes, mini vacations, and so on. Use small rewards for motivation while in training. Save a large reward for after completing the 5K, 10K, or half-marathon. This reward will be very motivating on race day!

Time-Based Goals

Set a date or time frame that you will achieve your goal. This helps prevent procrastination.

Example

Not Time-Based: "I want to walk a half-marathon."

Time-Based: "I want to walk the half-marathon in Indianapolis on May 7."

Keep in mind that goal setting is ongoing—once you achieve a goal, set another one. For example, once you complete your 10K, consider what you want to achieve next—possibly another 10K, another 10K at a faster pace, a half-marathon, a triathlon, and so on. The subsequent goal setting does not need to occur at the finish line of the race, but it should happen within weeks following the race to keep the fitness ball rolling.

What Are Your Goals?

In this section, you will have the opportunity to reflect on your goals and define them more specifically through the establishment of short, intermediate, and long-term goals. As an example, consider two commonly held goals in relation to training for a 5K, 10K, or half-marathon:

- Increase overall fitness
- Successfully complete the race distance

These goals can be broken down into short, intermediate, and long-term goals as well as their connection to specific training considerations.

A common goal is to increase fitness. This should be the primary goal for first time exercisers. Your secondary goal should be to complete the 5K, 10K, or half-marathon. This will help you stay motivated to exercise and get fit first. Keep the intensity low and enjoyable. Consistency is the key to success. Examples of short, intermediate, and long-term goals for individuals who want to increase their fitness might include:

- Short-term goal: "I will walk three times a week at a low-moderate intensity."
- Intermediate goal: "I will walk the 10K at a comfortable pace in order to finish successfully."
- Long-term goal: "I will look for another 10K or half-marathon to train for after the successful completion of my first 10K."

The second common goal is, "I just want to finish!" This is a common goal for individuals who have been exercising regularly but have never attempted a walking or running race, especially the longer distances. If this is your primary goal, focus on staying injury free by keeping the intensity low most of the time. Try to keep up with the long run/walk mileage as it increases and do not try to run/walk through injury. Speedwork or faster-paced training is not recommended. Your 5K, 10K, or half-marathon pace should be at a comfortable to moderate level. Examples of short, intermediate, and long-term goals for individuals who want to successfully complete a 5K, 10K, or half-marathon might include the following:

- Short-term goal: "I will run three times a week at a low-moderate intensity, plus three days a week of cross training."
- Intermediate goal: "I will successfully complete each long run scheduled during my training for the half-marathon to adequately prepare for the race."

■ Long-term goal: "I will run two half-marathons a year (in the spring and fall) for the next two years."

Now is your chance to document your short, intermediate, and long-term health and fitness goals. What do you want to accomplish?

What Are Your Short-Term Goals?

Short-term goals are your objectives that can be accomplished in a very short amount of time, such as a weekly or daily goal. An example of an appropriate short-term goal is, "I will run three times this week for 20 minutes each time."

Document three of your short-term goals:

1.

2.

3.

What Are Your Intermediate Goals?

Intermediate goals are objectives that can be accomplished in a somewhat lengthy amount of time, such as several months. An example of an appropriate intermediate goal is, "I will train for the half-marathon for the next three to four months and will complete the entire 13.1 miles."

Document three of your intermediate goals:

1.

2.

3.

What Are Your Long-Term Goals?

Long-term goals are objectives that can be accomplished down the road, such as one to three years in the future. An example of an appropriate long-term goal is, "I will run a 10K race each year for the next three years and improve my time each year."

Document three of your long-term goals:

1.

2.

3.

How Are You Going to Accomplish Your Goals?

After contemplating and documenting your short, intermediate, and long-term goals, you need to consider what needs to be done to make your goals a reality. This next step forces you to consider an action plan of *how* you are going to accomplish your goals.

How Are You Going to Accomplish Your Short-Term Goals?

Using the short-term goal example from the last section, an action plan for ensuring success in accomplishing the goal would be, "I plan to get up a half hour earlier and run before work three days this week."

What is your action plan for making each of your short-term goals a reality?

1.

2.

3.

How Are You Going to Accomplish Your Intermediate Goals?

Using the intermediate goal example from the last section, an action plan for ensuring success in accomplishing the goal would be, "I plan to increase my mileage weekly and build endurance."

What is your action plan for making each of your intermediate goals a reality?

1.

2.

3.

How Are You Going to Accomplish Your Long-Term Goals?

Using the long-term goal example from the last section, an action plan for ensuring success in accomplishing the goal would be, "I will make running a permanent part of my lifestyle."

What is your action plan for making each of your long-term goals a reality?

1.

2.

3.

What Obstacles Might You Encounter in Your Quest to Accomplish Your Goals?

Even the best-laid plans can be disrupted by unexpected life events. Consider your main action plan for achieving your goals and then anticipate the obstacles or barriers that might prevent you from being successful. Once you realize what might become a stumbling block, you can develop your back-up plan of how to overcome those barriers so that in the end, you will ultimately be successful.

In the following space, contemplate and then document the obstacles that might prevent you from achieving your short, intermediate, and long-term goals, as well as your proposed solutions to overcoming those obstacles.

Short-term goals

Anticipated obstacles	*Proposed solutions*
1a.	1b.
2a.	2b.
3a.	3b.

Intermediate goals

Anticipated obstacles	*Proposed solutions*
1a.	1b.
2a.	2b.
3a.	3b.

Long-term goals

Anticipated obstacles	*Proposed solutions*
1a.	1b.
2a.	2b.
3a.	3b.

How Can You Track Your Progress?

After you have set short, intermediate, and long-term goals, track your progress toward your goals. Documenting your weekly exercise and daily nutrition will help you stay focused each day and can serve as a great motivation tool to see how far you have come. You can keep a log in several different ways—on a calendar, in a daily planner, in a spiral notebook, or on structured log sheets. This book provides tear-out training and nutrition log sheets for you in the appendix to help you track your progress toward the successful completion of a 5K, 10K, or half-marathon.

How Can You Use the Training Logs in This Book?

Our training logs, shown in Figures 2.1 and 2.2, allow you to record workout information related to the following:

- *Date*—Recording the date will allow you to see your progression over time as well as to ensure you are keeping on track with the 5K, 10K, or half-marathon protocols presented in this book. With busy lives, it is easy to forget how long it has been since your last long walk/run, when you last performed a cross training session, and so on. Tracking the date will also allow you to compare how you are progressing at the same time next year.

- *Duration*—The length of time it takes to complete a walk, run, or cross training session is required to establish your current pace. If you have a goal of walking or running a race at a specific minute/mile pace, you must know the average time it takes you to complete a mile. For example, suppose your goal is to run a 10 minute/mile pace during a 10K. In your first week of training, you completed three miles in 30:18. In this initial run, your pace was 10:06 (30:18 minutes ÷ 3 miles = 10:06 minute/mile). Therefore, you are close to your goal and after several weeks of training, a 10 minute/mile pace is manageable and realistic. However, if your goal was to run the 10K in an 8 minute/mile pace, it might be wise to re-evaluate your goal and strive for the 8 minute/mile pace within the next two to three years.

- *Distance*—How far you have gone in one walk/run or the entire week is critical information. The only way you will be able to determine if you are following the "5%–10% Rule" (do not increase your mileage by more than 5%–10% each week) is if you record your total distance and tabulate the change each week. For example, if you walked 10 miles one week, you should not walk more than 11 miles the following week [{10 miles + (10 miles × 10%)} = 10 miles + 1 mile = 11 miles].

- *Heart rate*—Heart rate is a measure of your exercise intensity. In the next chapter you will determine your easy, moderate, and hard heart rate training zones. Keeping track of your heart rate each day will help ensure that you are challenging yourself enough to improve and meet your goals, but not overdoing it, which can lead to fatigue and injury.

- *Outside temperature and humidity*—Environmental factors can dramatically affect your walk or run. It is important to understand how your body reacts to different weather conditions so you are prepared on race day for wind, rain, snow, or heat. You will find that your heart rate, walking or running pace, perceived effort levels, and hydration needs will vary greatly based on environmental temperatures and humidity levels.

■ *Comments*—This section is perfect for recording what type of workout you completed (that is, walking, running, cross training session, and so on), your minute/mile pace, how you were feeling, the course description, or who you exercised with that day. When you look back to review your logs, the Comments section helps you to remember where you were, what you were doing, and why you performed the way you did.

Figure 2.1 shows a sample training log. However, do not forget that your weekly tear-our training logs are in the appendix of this book. Figure 2.2 shows a sample training log that includes documentation of all the information discussed previously.

FIGURE 2.1

Sample blank training log.

TRAINING LOG

MONDAY				
DATE	DURATION	DISTANCE	HEART RATE	TEMP
COMMENTS (i.e. type of exercise; pace):				

TUESDAY				
DATE	DURATION	DISTANCE	HEART RATE	TEMP
COMMENTS (i.e. type of exercise; pace):				

WEDNESDAY				
DATE	DURATION	DISTANCE	HEART RATE	TEMP
COMMENTS (i.e. type of exercise; pace):				

THURSDAY				
DATE	DURATION	DISTANCE	HEART RATE	TEMP
COMMENTS (i.e. type of exercise; pace):				

FRIDAY				
DATE	DURATION	DISTANCE	HEART RATE	TEMP
COMMENTS (i.e. type of exercise; pace):				

SATURDAY				
DATE	DURATION	DISTANCE	HEART RATE	TEMP
COMMENTS (i.e. type of exercise; pace):				

SUNDAY				
DATE	DURATION	DISTANCE	HEART RATE	TEMP
COMMENTS (i.e. type of exercise; pace):				

SUMMARY		
WEEK'S TOTAL	MONTH'S TOTAL	YEAR'S TOTAL
LONGEST RUN-WALK	SHORTEST RUN-WALK	AVERAGE RUN-WALK

How Can You Use the Nutrition Logs in This Book?

Use nutrition logs to record your dietary information related to the following:

■ *Meals and snacks*—Nutrition is a vital component to training for a 5K, 10K, or half-marathon. Without the proper timing of quality fluid and fuel, your body will not be able to reach its potential. Recording your meals and snacks each day will bring an awareness of the types, quantities, and timing of foods eaten and how it affects your walking and running. Later in this book we will discuss the nutrition guidelines for your daily training diet as well as recommendations for race day. A food record will allow you to analyze what you are currently eating and drinking and determine what adjustments need to be made.

FIGURE 2.2

Sample training
log.

TRAINING LOG

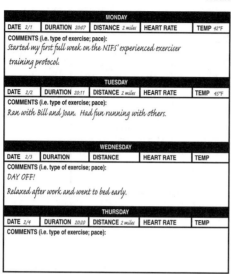
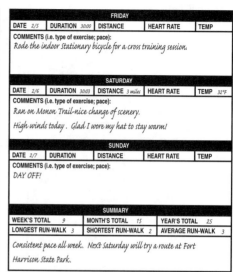

Serving sizes and total servings per day—In order to determine if you are eating enough, too little, or too much, you must be familiar with serving sizes and how many servings from each food group you should consume in a day to meet your overall needs. Keep in mind that a typical American "serving" is usually much larger than a "serving" as suggested by the Food Guide Pyramid; many people perceive one serving as a plateful, which can actually be multiple servings as defined by the Food Guide Pyramid. It is helpful if you measure your foods while preparing meals to be more accurate in your dietary record keeping.

Goals for the week—This section allows you to maintain focus on your nutrition habits while training for a 5K, 10K, or half-marathon. Oftentimes, walkers and runners develop tunnel vision while training, which can cause people to neglect other areas of their lives, such as their daily nutrition. Goals should be small and manageable for a one-week time span. Goals can consist of ways to change and adapt, or habits that you want to solidify by practicing.

A sample nutrition log is presented in Figure 2.3. Similar to the training logs, the appendix of this book contains weekly tear-out nutrition logs for your use during your 5K, 10K, or half-marathon training. A sample day is posted at the top of each log to provide guidance and act as a reminder of how to record and track your daily food and beverage consumption.

FIGURE 2.3

Sample nutrition log.

NUTRITION LOGS

Goals for the week: _____

		BREAKFAST	LUNCH	DINNER	SNACKS
SAMPLE	Sugar- [XX] -Fat Meat- [XX] [XX] -Milk [SERVINGS] Vegetable- [XXX] [X] -Fruit Grain- [XXX] [XXXXXX]	• 2 slices of whole wheat toast (2 grains) • 1 t margarine (1 fat) • banana (1 fruit) • 6 oz. orange juice (1 fruit)	• Chicken Caesar Salad – 2 oz. grilled chicken (1 meat) – 2 cups mixed greens (2 veg.) – 1 tb. caesar dressing (1 fat) • 2 breadsticks (2 grains) • 1 cup yogurt (1 milk)	• 3 oz. grilled chicken (1 meat) • 1/2 cup cooked brown rice (1 grain) • 1 t margarine (1 fat) • 1/2 cup cooked broccoli (1 veg.) • 8 oz. skim milk (1 milk)	• 1 oz. mini pretzels (1 grain) • 2 chocolate chip cookies (2 fat) • 6 oz. grape fruit juice (1 fruit)
MONDAY	Sugar- -Fat Meat- -Milk [SERVINGS] Vegetable- -Fruit Grain-				
TUESDAY	Sugar- -Fat Meat- -Milk [SERVINGS] Vegetable- -Fruit Grain-				
WEDNESDAY	Sugar- -Fat Meat- -Milk [SERVINGS] Vegetable- -Fruit Grain-				

NUTRITION LOGS

Goals for the week: _____

		BREAKFAST	LUNCH	DINNER	SNACKS
THURSDAY	Sugar- -Fat Meat- -Milk [SERVINGS] Vegetable- -Fruit Grain-				
FRIDAY	Sugar- -Fat Meat- -Milk [SERVINGS] Vegetable- -Fruit Grain-				
SATURDAY	Sugar- -Fat Meat- -Milk [SERVINGS] Vegetable- -Fruit Grain-				
SUNDAY	Sugar- -Fat Meat- -Milk [SERVINGS] Vegetable- -Fruit Grain-				

THE ABSOLUTE MINIMUM

- If you are a first-time exerciser, make an appointment with your doctor to gain medical clearance before beginning the 5K, 10K, or half-marathon training programs presented in this book.

- Consider scheduling a fitness assessment to obtain valuable information on your current fitness level, which can provide incentive for improvements over the course of the training program.

- Establish S.M.A.R.T. short, intermediate, and long-term goals to stay focused and motivated.

- Track your progress toward your goals by using the tear-out training and nutrition logs located in the appendix of this book.

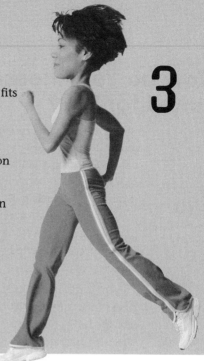

3

CHOOSING YOUR PROGRAM

Let the training begin!

Now that you have set your goals in Chapter 2, "Getting Started," it is time to determine the training protocol to help you achieve those goals. There are three different protocols presented in this chapter for 5K, 10K, and half-marathon distances: *fitness walking*, *run/walk*, and *experienced exerciser*. An explanation of the protocols will guide you in choosing the program ideally suited for your needs, goals, and current abilities. Each protocol will dictate the frequency, duration, and intensity of your exercise sessions. To allow you to fully understand how to monitor your intensity while walking, running, or cross training, this chapter will also review training heart rate ranges and the rating of perceived exertion scale. The final section will examine the importance of cross training and provide examples of how to include cross training in your weekly routine. Choose your protocol wisely and make sure to have fun!

How Do You Choose the Program That Is Best Suited for You?

In the last chapter, you established goals. Now it is time to determine how you can make these goals a reality by choosing the training program that best fits your needs. Based on whether your goal is to complete a 5K, 10K, or half-marathon, make a decision between these three training protocols: fitness walking, run/walk, or experienced exerciser. Be conservative when choosing a program so you can reach your goals safely and without injury. Base this decision on your current fitness level and regular exercise routine. To help you choose the right program, detailed descriptions of each protocol are provided in this section.

The three different 5K training protocols are all 8 weeks in length, the 10K protocols are 11 weeks, and the half-marathon protocols are 15 weeks. Based on the date of the race you choose to complete, count backwards from the race to know when you are to begin your training. *Do not* rush your training and jump into one of the training protocols at week 2, 4, 6, and so on regardless of the length of the race. Plan ahead to make sure you have plenty of time to successfully complete the entire training program to prevent injuries or health complications. If you just started reading this book and your planned race is a couple of weeks away, choose a later race that will allow you to train appropriately by completing the entire training program.

The three different training protocols (fitness walking, run/walk, and experienced exerciser) for each distance (5K, 10K, and half-marathon) assume that your long walk or run of the week will be on Saturdays. If this is not a convenient day for you, shift the protocol so you are completing the long workout on a day when you are not rushed by work or other commitments. However, maintain the spacing of the workouts

note

I am sure you are eager to begin your training. However, it is critical that you are conservative when choosing your 5K, 10K, or half-marathon protocol. Pushing yourself too hard can lead to injury and prevent you from achieving your goals.

caution

Do not try to condense the protocols to rush through your training. Each program is designed to allow for an appropriate progression of time or mileage in preparation for your 5K, 10K, or half-marathon race as well as for rest and recovery throughout the program. Skipping weeks by starting late can lead to fatigue and injury.

to allow for rest and recovery. For example, shifting the long workout to Sunday will cause the entire protocol to shift by one day.

Please read through each protocol description before deciding on your best option. Choose wisely and have fun! If you go to http://www.quepublishing.com and type this book's ISBN (0789733145) into the Search field to go to this book's web page, you will find printable PDF versions of all of these protocols available for download.

Is a "Fitness Walking" Protocol Right for You?

The Fitness Walking protocols are geared for the fitness walker who is walking one to three days per week, or the first-time exerciser. The program is based on time rather than mileage. It is designed to increase your fitness level as well as help you successfully complete your 5K, 10K, or half-marathon. These protocols schedule only three days a week of exercise, which is ideal for first-time exercisers. Your focus should be on the long walk of the week while including two additional days of walking or cross training at an easy or moderate pace. The following list describes additional program characteristics:

- The Fitness Walking protocols are appropriate for you if your goals are to increase aerobic fitness and to finish the 5K, 10K, or half-marathon.
- Consider your current fitness level. You must be able to walk at least one or two miles comfortably at a 16–20 minute/mile pace.
- The Fitness Walking protocols include two to three walking workouts per week with one optional cross training session. The intensity is easy to moderate.

Figure 3.1 through 3.3 show the Fitness Walking protocols for the 5K, 10K, and half-marathon races.

FIGURE 3.1

5K Fitness Walking protocol.

5K - Fitness Walking (~20 minute/mile walk pace)								
	Rest Day	Easy or CT	Rest Day	Moderate	Rest Day	Long	Rest Day	
Week	Monday	Tuesday	Wednesday	Thursday	Friday	Saturday	Sunday	TOTAL TIME
1		0:20:00		0:20:00		0:20:00		1:00:00
2		0:20:00		0:20:00		0:30:00		1:10:00
3		0:20:00		0:20:00		0:40:00		1:20:00
4		0:20:00		0:20:00		0:20:00		1:00:00
5		0:20:00		0:20:00		0:50:00		1:30:00
6		0:20:00		0:20:00		1:00:00		1:40:00
7		0:20:00		0:20:00		0:30:00		1:10:00
8		0:20:00		0:10:00		Race Day - 5K		1:32:00

FIGURE 3.2

10K Fitness Walking protocol.

10K - Fitness Walking (~18 minutes/mile walk pace)								
	Rest Day	Easy or CT	Rest Day	Moderate	Rest Day	Long	Rest Day	
Week	Monday	Tuesday	Wednesday	Thursday	Friday	Saturday	Sunday	TOTAL TIME
1		0:20:00		0:20:00		0:30:00		1:10:00
2		0:20:00		0:20:00		0:40:00		1:20:00
3		0:20:00		0:20:00		0:50:00		1:30:00
4		0:20:00		0:20:00		0:30:00		1:10:00
5		0:20:00		0:20:00		1:00:00		1:40:00
6		0:20:00		0:20:00		1:10:00		1:50:00
7		0:20:00		0:20:00		0:40:00		1:20:00
8		0:20:00		0:20:00		1:20:00		2:00:00
9		0:20:00		0:20:00		1:40:00		2:20:00
10		0:20:00		0:20:00		0:30:00		1:10:00
11		0:20:00		0:20:00		Race Day - 10K		2:31:00

FIGURE 3.3

Half-marathon Fitness Walking protocol.

Week	Rest Day Monday	Moderate or CT Tuesday	Rest Day/Easy Wednesday	Easy Thursday	Rest Day Friday	Long Saturday	Rest Day Sunday	TOTAL TIME
1		0:20:00		0:20:00		0:30:00		1:10:00
2		0:20:00		0:20:00		0:50:00		1:30:00
3		0:20:00		0:20:00		1:00:00		1:40:00
4		0:20:00		0:20:00		0:40:00		1:20:00
5		0:20:00		0:20:00		1:10:00		1:50:00
6		0:20:00		0:20:00		1:20:00		2:00:00
7		0:20:00		0:20:00		1:40:00		2:20:00
8		0:20:00		0:20:00		0:50:00		1:30:00
9		0:20:00		0:20:00		2:00:00		2:40:00
10		0:20:00		0:20:00		2:20:00		3:00:00
11			0:30:00			0:30:00		1:00:00
12		0:20:00		0:20:00		2:50:00		3:30:00
13			0:50:00			0:50:00		1:40:00
14		0:30:00		0:20:00		0:30:00		1:20:00
15		0:20:00		0:20:00		Race Day - Half Marathon		4:10:00

Use the following workout key for these protocols:

■ EASY—Keep intensity low and at a conversational level.

Intensity should be within 50%–70% of your Target Heart Rate or 11–12 on the RPE scale.

■ MODERATE—Slightly more difficult than easy.

Intensity should be within 75%–85% of your Target Heart Range or 13–14 on the RPE scale.

■ LONG—Keep intensity low and at a conversational level. Focus on completing the distance.

Intensity should be within 50%–70% of your Target Heart Range or 11–12 on the RPE scale.

■ CT (Cross Train)—Workout for the designed amount of time on aerobic or strength equipment. Keep intensity low to moderate.

Is a "Run/Walk" Protocol Right for You?

This program is designed for first-time walkers, runners, and those who want to follow a combination run/walk training regimen. This program is based on mileage instead of time with the exception of your cross training day that is scheduled in time instead of miles. If you are interested in following the run/walk regimen, the mileage in all three race lengths will be completed by alternating running for three minutes and walking for one minute. The combination run/walk regimen is perfect if you are interested in transitioning from walking to running while staying injury free. This protocol increases the number of days of exercise to four: three days of walking, running, or run/walking (including one long workout), plus a cross training day. Below are additional program characteristics:

- The Run/Walk protocols are appropriate for you if your goals are to increase fitness levels through regular walking, running, or a combination of walking and running; and to finish the 5K, 10K, or half-marathon race.

- Consider your current fitness level. You must be able to walk, run, or run/walk one to two miles comfortably. No requirements on speed.

- The mileage in the Run/Walk protocols range from 3–6 miles per week for the 5K program up to 6–18 miles per week for the half-marathon program. The intensity is easy to moderate.

Figures 3.4 through 3.6 show the Run/Walk protocols for the 5K, 10K, and half-marathon races.

FIGURE 3.4

5K Run/Walk protocol.

5K - Run/Walk	Run/walk regimen option: Alternate running for 3 minutes and walking for 1 minute for easy, moderate and long workouts							
Week	CT Monday	Easy Tuesday	Rest Day Wednesday	Moderate Thursday	Rest Day Friday	Long Saturday	Rest Day Sunday	TOTAL MILEAGE
1	0:30:00	1		1		1		3
2	0:30:00	1		1		2		4
3	0:30:00	2		1		3		6
4	0:30:00	2		2		2		6
5	0:30:00	2		2		3		7
6	0:30:00	2		2		4		8
7	0:30:00	2		2		2		6
8	0:20:00	2		1		Race Day - 5K		6.1

FIGURE 3.5

10K Run/Walk protocol.

10K - Run/Walk	Run/walk regimen option: Alternate running for 3 minutes and walking for 1 minute for easy, moderate and long workouts							
Week	CT Monday	Easy Tuesday	Rest Day Wednesday	Moderate Thursday	Rest Day Friday	Long Saturday	Rest Day Sunday	TOTAL MILEAGE
1	0:30:00	2		2		2		6
2	0:30:00	2		2		3		7
3	0:30:00	2		2		4		8
4	0:30:00	2		2		2		6
5	0:30:00	2		2		4		8
6	0:30:00	2		2		3		7
7	0:30:00	2		2		5		9
8	0:30:00	2		2		3		7
9	0:30:00	2		2		6		10
10	0:30:00	2		2		3		7
11	0:20:00	2		2		Race Day - 10K		10.2

FIGURE 3.6

Half-marathon Run/Walk protocol.

Half Marathon - Run/Walk	Run/walk regimen option: Alternate running for 3 minutes and walking for 1 minute for easy, moderate and long workouts							
Week	CT Monday	Easy Tuesday	Rest Day Wednesday	Moderate Thursday	Rest Day Friday	Long Saturday	Rest Day Sunday	TOTAL MILEAGE
1	0:30:00	2		2		2		6
2	0:30:00	2		2		3		7
3	0:30:00	2		2		3		7
4	0:30:00	3		2		4		9
5	0:30:00	3		2		3		8
6	0:30:00	3		2		5		10
7	0:30:00	3		2		7		12
8	0:30:00	3		3		4		10
9	0:30:00	3		3		8		14
10	0:30:00	3		3		9		15
11	0:30:00	3		3		4		10
12	0:30:00	3		3		10		16
13	0:30:00	3		3		12		18
14	0:30:00	3		3		3		9
15		3		2		Race Day - Half Marathon		18.1

Use the following workout key for these protocols:

- EASY—Keep intensity low and at a conversational level.

  Intensity should be within 50%–70% of your Target Heart Rate or 11–12 on the RPE scale.

- MODERATE—Slightly more difficult than easy.

  Intensity should be within 75%–85% of your Target Heart Range or 13–14 on the RPE scale.

- LONG—Keep intensity low and at a conversational level. Focus on completing the distance.

  Intensity should be within 50%–70% of your Target Heart Range or 11–12 on the RPE scale.

- CT (Cross Train)—Work out for the designed amount of time on aerobic or strength equipment. Keep intensity low to moderate.

Is an "Experienced Exerciser" Protocol Right for You?

The Experienced Exerciser program is designed for individuals who have been regularly active but not necessarily focused on walking or running. This is a mileage-based protocol (with cross training days listed in time) and is appropriate for either walkers or runners. Similar to the Fitness Walking and Run/Walk programs, the emphasis is on the long walk or run, which will condition you to comfortably and safely complete the 3.1, 6.2, or 13.1 miles of your goal race. Most of your weekly mileage should be completed at an intensity that is easy and comfortable, with one moderate-intensity workout per week. The programs include 3–4 days of walking or running and 1–2 days of cross training so you can continue to enjoy your other favorite activities.

- The Experienced Exerciser protocols are appropriate if your goals are to increase fitness with the challenge of a new activity/sport and to finish your 5K, 10K, or half-marathon.

- Consider your current fitness level. You must be able to walk or run at least two to three miles comfortably. No requirements on speed.

- The mileage in the Experienced Exerciser protocols range from 6–9 miles per week for the 5K program up to 9–21 miles per week for the half-marathon program.

FIGURE 3.7

5K Experienced Exerciser protocol.

5K - Experienced Exerciser								
	CT	Easy	Rest Day	Moderate	CT	Long	Rest Day	
Week	Monday	Tuesday	Wednesday	Thursday	Friday	Saturday	Sunday	TOTAL MILEAGE
1	0:30:00	2		2	0:30:00	2		6
2	0:30:00	2		2	0:30:00	3		7
3	0:30:00	2		2	0:30:00	3		7
4	0:30:00	2		2	0:30:00	2		6
5	0:30:00	3		2	0:30:00	3		8
6	0:30:00	3		2	0:30:00	4		9
7	0:30:00	3		2	0:30:00	2		7
8	0:20:00	2		1		Race Day - 5K		6.1

FIGURE 3.8

10K Experienced Exerciser protocol.

10K - Experienced Exerciser								
	CT	Moderate	Rest Day	Easy	CT	Long	Rest Day	
Week	Monday	Tuesday	Wednesday	Thursday	Friday	Saturday	Sunday	TOTAL MILEAGE
1	0:30:00	2		2	0:30:00	2		6
2	0:30:00	2		2	0:30:00	3		7
3	0:30:00	2		2	0:30:00	4		8
4	0:30:00	2		2	0:30:00	2		6
5	0:30:00	3		2	0:30:00	4		9
6	0:30:00	3		2	0:30:00	5		10
7	0:30:00	3		2	0:30:00	3		8
8	0:30:00	3		2	0:30:00	5		10
9	0:30:00	3		2	0:30:00	6		11
10	0:30:00	3		2	0:30:00	3		8
11	0:20:00	2		2		Race Day - 10K		10.2

FIGURE 3.9

Half-marathon Experienced Exerciser protocol.

Half Marathon - Experienced Exerciser								
	Easy	Moderate	Rest Day	Easy	CT	Long	Rest Day	
Week	Monday	Tuesday	Wednesday	Thursday	Friday	Saturday	Sunday	TOTAL MILEAGE
1	2	2		2	0:30:00	3		9
2	2	2		2	0:30:00	4		10
3	2	3		2	0:30:00	4		11
4	2	3		2	0:30:00	5		12
5	2	4		2	0:30:00	6		14
6	2	3		2	0:30:00	5		12
7	3	4		2	0:30:00	7		16
8	3	3		2	0:30:00	8		16
9	3	4		2	0:30:00	5		14
10	3	3		2	0:30:00	9		17
11	3	4		2	0:30:00	10		19
12	3	3		2	0:30:00	6		14
13	3	4		2	0:30:00	12		21
14	3	3		2	0:30:00	3		11
15		3		2		Race Day - Half Marathon		18.1

Use the following workout key for these protocols:

- EASY—Keep intensity low and at a conversational level.

  Intensity should be within 50%–70% of your Target Heart Rate or 11–12 on the RPE scale.

- MODERATE—Slightly more difficult than easy.

  Intensity should be within 75%–85% of your Target Heart Range or 13–14 on the RPE scale.

- LONG—Keep intensity low and at a conversational level. Focus on completing the distance.

  Intensity should be within 50%–70% of your Target Heart Range or 11–12 on the RPE scale.

- CT (Cross Train)—Work out for the designed amount of time on aerobic or strength equipment. Keep intensity low to moderate.

How Can You Determine Exercise Intensity?

Each training protocol within this book refers to "easy" or "moderate" intensity walks or runs throughout the week. It is critical that you understand what easy and moderate actually mean as well as how they feel in order to train appropriately. Two ways to determine exercise intensity are by calculating your target heart rate ranges and subjectively measuring your rating of perceived exertion while walking and running.

Measuring your heart rate during exercise provides an objective measure of your exercise intensity. Monitoring your heart rate is an excellent tool to determine more precisely how hard you are working so you can actually walk or run "easy" on your easy days and "moderate" on your moderate days. If you relate best to numbers and exact measurements, monitoring your heart rate may be a good option for you. However, you must realize that heart rates can vary daily based on sleep patterns, stress levels, hydration status, or the ingestion of medications. Therefore, it is best to use heart rate in combination with your rating of perceived exertion.

The *rating of perceived exertion* (RPE) is a psychophysical scale developed to have a high correlation with heart rates and other metabolic parameters. The RPE scale subjectively measures exercise intensity by using verbal expressions to evaluate the perception of effort during walking or running. The RPE scale is an excellent tool to use if you are not a numbers person or do not want to be bothered with monitoring your heart rate during exercise. Ideally, you will use the RPE scale in conjunction with heart rate monitoring during exercise. Using both methods will confirm you are walking or running at an appropriate intensity. For example, if you are completing an easy day of exercise and your heart rate is within your calculated easy range but it feels moderate or hard, this is an indication that you are tired and you need to decrease the intensity of your walk or run by slowing the pace. Another example might be that you are completing a moderate workout and your heart rate is within your moderate intensity range, but it feels easy. In this case, you might push the pace a little more to achieve a moderate level of perceived exertion.

The next section reviews how to establish your target heart rate ranges, explains how to use the rating of perceived exertion, and finally, discusses the relationship between heart rate, RPE, and walking or running pace.

How Can You Establish Your Target Heart Rate Ranges?

Determining and training within various heart rate ranges can help to improve fitness, enhance performance, and prevent injury and overtraining. The following formulas, collectively titled the Karvonen Formula developed by Dr. M. Karvonen, will lead you through the process of calculating your Target Heart Rate Ranges. Each protocol within this book refers to easy or moderate days of training, with all long workouts performed at an easy intensity. None of the protocols incorporate "hard" intensity workouts. For beginners, training at too high of an intensity can lead to injuries. You will calculate your "hard" heart rate range solely for the purpose of recognizing when you are working too hard and therefore need to slow down in order to decrease your exercise intensity.

Calculating your target heart rate ranges requires the knowledge of two variables: your *maximum heart rate* and your *resting heart rate.* Your maximum heart rate, or the greatest number of beats per minute your heart can pump during exercise, can be directly measured during a maximal effort treadmill test or through an estimation equation. The results of a treadmill test are extremely accurate; however, the test can be costly, time-intensive, and risky for some individuals. The estimation equation is quick and easy; however, the results have been shown to be highly variable as compared to actual measurements and therefore can be somewhat inaccurate. For beginners, using the maximum heart rate estimation equation will be sufficient in providing a ballpark figure to aim for during walking and running. If you choose to continue walking and running, and you desire more precise training heart rate ranges, you can inquire about scheduling a maximal effort treadmill test with your physician or fitness specialist.

The target heart rate range calculations use the maximum heart rate estimation equation and resting heart rate measurements. The only variable in the maximum heart rate range estimation equation is age. In general, as we age, our maximum heart rate will decline. For the target heart rate range calculation, you are also required to measure your resting heart rate on three separate occasions. Your resting heart rate is the number of times your heart beats per minute while at rest. It is best to take your resting heart rate first thing in the morning—before getting out of bed, having coffee, or going to the bathroom—by counting your pulse for one full minute. Your pulse can be found at your carotid artery in your neck, just off center, or on the inside of your wrist, just below your thumb, by using your two fore fingers. You should not use your thumb to measure your heart rate because it has a pulse of its own. After recording your resting heart rate for three days, take the average of the three measurements.

Use the following blanks to enter your numbers. If you are confused by any part of these Karvonen Formula calculations, refer to the sample calculations later in this chapter.

1. Maximal Heart Rate (220 – your age) = _____

2. Average of Resting Heart Rate for three days (taken first thing in the morning):

   Day 1 _____ Day 2 _____ Day 3 _____

   Average of 3 days = _____

3. Maximal Heart Rate minus Average Resting Heart Rate = Heart Rate Reserve (HRR)

   _____ – _____ = _____ (HRR)

4. Training Intensity Range (Heart Rate Reserve × 50%–96%):

   Easy

   (HRR × 0.50) = _____ × 0.50 = _____ beats/minute

   (HRR × 0.70) = _____ × 0.70 = _____ beats/minute

   Moderate

   (HRR × 0.75) = _____ × 0.75 = _____ beats/minute

   (HRR × 0.85) = _____ × 0.85 = _____ beats/minute

   Hard

   (HRR × 0.86) = _____ × 0.86 = _____ beats/minute

   (HRR × 0.96) = _____ × 0.96 = _____ beats/minute

5. Add the Average Resting Heart Rate to the Training Intensity Range to find your Target Heart Rate Range.

   Easy

   _____ + (_____ – _____) = _____ – _____ beats/minute

   Moderate

   _____ + (_____ – _____) = _____ – _____ beats/minute

   Hard

   _____ + (_____ – _____) = _____ – _____ beats/minute

Sample Calculation

Susie is 45 years old.

1. Maximal Heart Rate (220 – age) = 220 – 45 = **175**

2. Average of Resting Heart Rate for 3 days (taken first thing in the morning):

   Day 1 = 75   Day 2 = 72   Day 3 = 76

   Average of 3 days = **74 beats per minute**

3. Maximal Heart Rate minus Average Resting Heart Rate = Heart Rate Reserve (HRR)

   175 – 74 = **101 beats per minute**

4. Training Intensity Range (Heart Rate Reserve × 50%–96%):

   Easy

   (HRR × 0.50) = 101 × 0.50 = **51 beats/minute**

   (HRR × 0.70) = 101 × 0.70 = **71 beats/minute**

   Moderate

   (HRR × 0.75) = 101 × 0.75 = **76 beats/minute**

   (HRR × 0.85) = 101 × 0.85 = **86 beats/minute**

   Hard

   (HRR × 0.86) = 101 × 0.86 = **87 beats/minute**

   (HRR × 0.96) = 101 × 0.96 = **97 beats/minute**

5. Add the Average Resting Heart Rate to the Training Intensity Range to find your Target Heart Rate Range.

   Easy

   74 + (51–71) = **125–145** beats/minute

   Moderate

   74 + (76–86) = **150–160** beats/minute

   Hard

   74 + (87–97) = **161–171** beats/minute

While walking or running, you can measure your heart rate by counting your pulse or wearing a heart rate monitor. Similar to measuring your resting rate heart, your pulse can be found at your carotid artery (neck) or your radial artery (wrist). The preferred location during exercise is at the radial artery. The reason for this preference is due to the presence of pressure receptors in your carotid artery. If too much pressure is applied to the neck while attempting to obtain an exercise heart rate, the body will sense an increased pressure in the arteries, causing a dilation of the blood vessels, which will decrease blood pressure and in turn possibly cause you to pass out. This is obviously not a desired result of taking your pulse while you are walking or running! Therefore, take your heart rate at your radial artery in your wrist. If counting your pulse is too challenging while you are exercising, consider purchasing a heart rate monitor. Wearing a heart rate monitor can make measuring your heart rate during exercise very easy and generally more accurate compared to counting your pulse with your fingers. Heart rate monitors can be purchased at most running/walking or sporting goods stores. For more information on heart rate monitors, see the following sidebar.

RUNNING AND WALKING TRAINING GADGETS—HEART RATE MONITORS

Monitoring your heart rate provides an objective measurement of your effort level during walking and running, ensuring you are working hard enough but not too hard. It can be challenging to accurately measure your own heart rate while walking and running. Therefore, heart rate monitors are an excellent tool for beginners as well as advanced exercisers. All heart rate monitors will include a watch-like receiver and a chest strap that detects your heart rate and sends the information to the receiver. Your heart rate is displayed continuously during your exercise session. All descriptions are taken directly from the products' websites.

Polar Heart Rate Monitor—M32 model (www.polarusa.com)—The M32 model includes the OwnCal™ feature, which counts the calories and fat you burn during an exercise session. It also includes the new OwnZone™ feature, which automatically determines each day's target heart rate zone. The M32 is a moderately priced model providing the essential components for the first-time walker or runner.

Timex Heart Rate Monitor—1440 Sport Digital model (www.timex.com)—For walkers and runners looking for an easy-to-use and inexpensive heart rate monitor, the Timex 1440 Sport Digital Heart Rate Monitor is an excellent choice. This model provides the basic features of a heart rate monitor without the bells and whistles of other models. The heart rate monitor can also be used as a stopwatch, allowing for the correlation between heart rate and walking/running pace.

NIKE Heart Rate Monitor—Imara model (www.nike.com)—This NIKE heart rate monitor features a calorie counter and programmable heart rate ranges. A moderately priced monitor, the Imara model is marketed specifically to women. Men can check out the more advanced, as well as more expensive, Triax Elite model.

How Can You Use the Rating of Perceived Exertion Scale?

The Borg Rating of Perceived Exertion (RPE) scale is a subjective measurement of exercise intensity. The original scale asks you to rate yourself from 6 (very, very light) to 20 (very, very hard) based on how you feel physically during exercise. The original scale was designed to directly correlate with heart rates measurements. Adding a zero to the end of each number on the RPE scale provides the corresponding heart rate. For example, a rating of 8 on the RPE would approximate a heart rate of 80. Newer scales use a 0–10 rating scale which many people find easier to relate to when providing a subjective measurement of exertion. Either scale is considered valid and useful. First-time walkers and runners should strive for an 11 (fairly light) to 15 (hard) on the 6–20 scale during exercise.

Use the RPE scale periodically during a walk or run to monitor your effort levels. Keep in mind when training for your first 5K, 10K, or half-marathon that a majority of your training should fall in the 11–13 range, with only a portion of one workout per week performed at a level of 14–15. Table 3.1 presents the Rating of Perceived Exertion Scale and the corresponding feelings in order to evaluate your exertion level during physical activity.

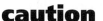

caution

Be careful to not work in the "hard" range of the RPE scale more than once a week during your training. To prevent injury and burnout, spend most of your time training in the "fairly light to somewhat hard" range of the RPE scale.

Table 3.1   Rating of Perceived Exertion During Activity

6	sitting (limited activity)
7	very, very light
8	
9	very light
10	
11	fairly light
12	
13	somewhat hard
14	
15	hard
16	
17	very hard
18	
19	very, very hard
20	total fatigue (exhaustion)

Source: Borg GAV. Med Sci Sports Exerc 14:377-387, 1982. Noble B., Borg GAV, Jacobs I., Ceci R., Kaiser P. Med Sci Sports Exerc 15:523-528, 1983

Can Pace Be Used in Conjunction with Heart Rate and RPE to Measure Walking and Running Intensity?

Your pace during one workout may not be a valid indicator of intensity because of the many variables that influence pace such as hills, wind, temperature, and so on. However, most walkers and runners find that over time they can identify specific paces that feel "easy" and paces that feel "hard." For most of your training for the 5K, 10K, or half-marathon, you want to find a pace that feels in the easy-to-moderate range of intensity. You can experiment with various walking and running paces, while measuring your heart rate or RPE to identify your easy and moderate pace ranges. Refer to the following Running and Walking Gadgets sidebar for information on a gadget that can help you monitor your pace no matter where you are walking or running—a GPS monitor.

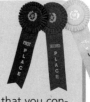

note

Set your goal for your 5K, 10K, or half-marathon finish time at a pace that you consider to be easy to moderate. The average pace you maintain for your long training walks and runs will give you a good indication of an appropriate pace for your race.

Figure 3.10 presents the total time to complete various distances from a 5K through a half-marathon for walkers and runners moving at a 6 minute per mile up to a 20 minute per mile pace. This chart is extremely useful for estimating your finish time for your 5K, 10K, or half-marathon goal race based on your current training pace.

RUNNING AND WALKING TRAINING GADGETS—GPS MONITORS

If you prefer to train according to pace and perceived exertion levels, a GPS (Global Positioning System) monitor may be the gadget for you. GPS monitors use a network of global positioning satellites to precisely track the distance and pace you are walking or running anywhere in the world. This is an excellent tool for individuals who travel frequently or walk or run in areas without marked paths. Product description taken directly from the Timex website.

Timex® Ironman Triathlon® Speed + Distance System (www.timex.com)—The Timex GPS device will track your distance and speed, providing essential information for training by pace. In addition, this model has a lap counter, timer, and separate weekday and weekend alarms. This device is also part of the Timex® Bodylink™ System, which can be used to measure your heart rate during workouts and record all data to be downloaded and tracked over time.

FIGURE 3.10

Walk/Run pace chart.

Distance (1K = 0.621 mile; 5K = 3.1 miles; 10K = 6.2 miles; 15K = 9.3 miles)

Mile Pace	5K	5 mile	10K	15K	10 mile	13.1 mile
6:00	18:38	30:00	37:16	55:54	1:00:00	1:18:36
6:15	19:25	31:15	38:49	58:14	1:02:30	1:21:52
6:30	20:11	32:30	40:22	1:00:34	1:05:00	1:25:09
6:45	20:58	33:45	41:56	1:02:53	1:07:30	1:28:26
7:00	21:44	35:00	43:29	1:05:13	1:10:00	1:31:42
7:15	22:31	36:15	45:02	1:07:33	1:12:30	1:34:59
7:30	23:18	37:30	46:35	1:09:53	1:15:00	1:38:15
7:45	24:04	38:45	48:08	1:12:12	1:17:30	1:41:32
8:00	24:51	40:00	49:41	1:14:32	1:20:00	1:44:48
8:15	25:37	41:15	51:15	1:16:52	1:22:30	1:48:05
8:30	26:24	42:30	52:48	1:19:12	1:25:00	1:51:21
8:45	27:10	43:45	54:21	1:21:31	1:27:30	1:54:38
9:00	27:57	45:00	55:54	1:23:51	1:30:00	1:57:54
9:15	28:44	46:15	57:27	1:26:11	1:32:30	2:01:11
9:30	29:30	47:30	59:00	1:28:31	1:35:00	2:04:27
9:45	30:17	48:45	1:00:34	1:30:50	1:37:30	2:07:44
10:00	31:03	50:00	1:02:07	1:33:10	1:40:00	2:11:00
10:15	31:50	51:15	1:03:40	1:35:30	1:42:30	2:14:17
10:30	32:37	52:30	1:05:13	1:37:50	1:45:00	2:17:33
10:45	33:23	53:45	1:06:46	1:40:09	1:47:30	2:20:50
11:00	34:10	55:00	1:08:19	1:42:29	1:50:00	2:24:06
11:15	34:56	56:15	1:09:53	1:44:49	1:52:30	2:27:23
11:30	35:43	57:30	1:11:26	1:47:09	1:55:00	2:30:39
11:45	36:29	58:45	1:12:59	1:49:28	1:57:30	2:33:56
12:00	37:16	1:00:00	1:14:32	1:51:48	2:00:00	2:37:12
12:15	38:03	1:01:15	1:16:05	1:54:08	2:02:30	2:40:29
12:30	38:49	1:02:30	1:17:38	1:56:28	2:05:00	2:43:45
12:45	39:36	1:03:45	1:19:12	1:58:47	2:07:30	2:47:02
13:00	40:22	1:05:00	1:20:45	2:01:07	2:10:00	2:50:18
13:15	41:09	1:06:15	1:22:18	2:03:27	2:12:30	2:53:34
13:30	41:56	1:07:30	1:23:51	2:05:47	2:15:00	2:56:51
13:45	42:42	1:08:45	1:25:24	2:08:06	2:17:30	3:00:07
14:00	43:29	1:10:00	1:26:57	2:10:26	2:20:00	3:03:24
14:15	44:15	1:11:15	1:28:31	2:12:46	2:22:30	3:06:40
14:30	45:02	1:12:30	1:30:04	2:15:06	2:25:00	3:09:57
14:45	45:48	1:13:45	1:31:37	2:17:25	2:27:30	3:13:13
15:00	46:35	1:15:00	1:33:10	2:19:45	2:30:00	3:16:30
15:15	47:22	1:16:15	1:34:43	2:22:05	2:32:30	3:19:46
15:30	48:08	1:17:30	1:36:16	2:24:25	2:35:00	3:23:03
15:45	48:55	1:18:45	1:37:50	2:26:44	2:37:30	3:26:19
16:00	49:41	1:20:00	1:39:23	2:29:04	2:40:00	3:29:36
16:15	50:28	1:21:15	1:40:56	2:31:24	2:42:30	3:32:52
16:30	51:15	1:22:30	1:42:29	2:33:44	2:45:00	3:36:09
16:45	52:01	1:23:45	1:44:02	2:36:03	2:47:30	3:39:25
17:00	52:48	1:25:00	1:45:35	2:38:23	2:50:00	3:42:42
17:15	53:34	1:26:15	1:47:09	2:40:43	2:52:30	3:45:58
17:30	54:21	1:27:30	1:48:42	2:43:03	2:55:00	3:49:15

What Is Cross Training and Why Is It Important?

All the protocols in this book recommend including a cross training session during each week of training. Cross training is any activity that does *not* include running or walking such as swimming, tennis, or weight lifting. These important workouts will help reduce impact stress, allow for recovery, add variety to your weekly exercise routine, and of course, improve your fitness by challenging your heart and muscles.

See Table 3.2 for more suggestions of activities to include on your cross training day.

Table 3.2   Suggestions for Cross Training

Basketball	Cycling
Elliptical trainers	Kickboxing
Pilates	Roller skating/blading
Swimming	Tai Chi
Tennis	Volleyball
Weight lifting	Yoga

Table 3.2 shows only a small sample of cross training activities—there are many, many more! Any activity that is different from walking or running counts as cross training.

before you head out the door

Know the prescribed intensity of your workout before beginning your walk or run and stick to it! If you want, wear a heart rate monitor or GPS monitor to track your intensity and pace. Remember, the RPE scale can be used at anytime and anywhere—no equipment required!

THE ABSOLUTE MINIMUM

- Be conservative when choosing a training protocol—find the one that fits your goals and current fitness level.
- Perform a majority, if not all, of your weekly workouts at an easy-to-moderate intensity to prevent injuries.
- Use both your target heart rate range and the RPE scale to monitor your intensity during walking and running.
- Over time, discover the correlation between various intensity levels and your walking or running pace.
- Incorporate at least one day of cross training into your weekly routine for variety, injury prevention, and fun!

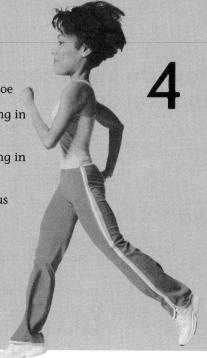

4

SAFETY PRECAUTIONS

Be serious about safety.

Walking and running are healthy for your heart, body, and mind. However, you are not exercising in your own little world; you need to be cognizant of what is going on around you to stay safe and healthy. Accidents are rare when walking and running outdoors, but when they do occur, the resulting injuries can be devastating. Mishaps can be as minor as a sprained ankle to as major as death. Therefore, be serious about staying safe. It is easy to do if you implement the guidelines in this chapter for finding the proper shoe fit, keeping cool in the summer and warm in the winter, as well as being aware of your surroundings and the presence of dogs, other animals, and people. So, put on the appropriate shoes, enjoy your walk/run, and as mom always told you, "Be safe."

How Do You Choose the Best Shoe for Running and Walking?

Walking into a running/walking or athletic store can be intimidating. There are so many types and brands of shoes to choose from, how do you know where to begin? The following seven clues will help to take the mystery out of buying the best running and walking shoes tailored to your needs and goals.

Clue #1: Fit, Fit, Fit

Shoes that fit properly are worth their weight in gold. The shoes that are right for your feet will feel like slippers, allowing you to "float on pillows" as you walk and run. Poorly fitting shoes can causing rubbing, bleeding, and blisters, which can stop you in your tracks because of pain and discomfort. Take your time finding the best shoes for your feet, and use the following guidelines:

- Find a shoe store that will measure your foot. Many people are surprised to learn that they are a half to one full size bigger or smaller than they thought.

- Because your feet expand while you run or walk, it is best to shop late in the day when your feet are at their widest and longest in size.

- Leave a thumb's width of room above the toes and in front of the toes. The toes should be able to move freely. An easy test is to bounce on the balls of your feet when trying on shoes; they should feel soft when you land, and your toes should move freely.

- Heel stability is important. The heel should be securely in place during all movement. If the rear foot slips up and down or side to side, the shoe is not giving enough support to the ankle and knee joints.

- Flared heels are important in walking and running where the initial contact occurs at the heel. The broader base shoe increases the surface area for the foot at contact. This helps provide a wide platform of support while at the same time dispersing impact over a wider surface area.

- Keep in mind that a proper fit is paramount in providing adequate support. The foot should feel supported without feeling restricted.

- Ask the salesperson if you can run or walk outside on the sidewalk or in the mall concourse when trying on different shoes.

Clue #2: Walking or Running Shoes? Which Is Best?

One of the most common questions asked of athletic shoe salespersons is which is best, a running shoe or a walking shoe. Walkers and runners can shop in the same store and both find the best fitting shoe. Walking-specific shoes are not as common as they once were because running shoes offer a greater variety of stability, cushion, and motion-control options. Walkers, do not be alarmed if a salesperson encourages you to buy a "running" shoe; it may in fact be the best option for you.

■ Walking shoes require more heel cushioning than front foot cushioning because your heel strikes the ground first. Walkers need a flexible shoe to allow for the toe-push off in their stride. A good running shoe is usually a good walking shoe.

■ Running shoes require adequate shock absorption because your feet are constantly pounding the ground. Proper arch and heel support (your heel should be snug in the back of the shoe) are needed. Flats can be advantageous in increasing speed. However, you should carefully consider the small gains in time before sacrificing the cushioning and support that results from running in flats. Heavy runners or heel strikers should avoid running in flats.

> **note**
>
> Ideally, runners should land on their forefoot, letting the heel drop slightly and then springing forward. Most runners land on their heels ("heel strikers") which can place more stress on the feet and up through the legs.

Clue #3: Shock Absorbency and Body Weight

Look for a shoe that offers the best shock absorbing materials to reduce the risk of impact injuries such as shin splints or stress fractures. Polyurethane provides excellent cushioning in the midsole to aid in shock absorbency. Many shoe companies are now using *nonfoam cushioning* (that is, honeycomb-shaped air cells) which is much more durable.

When you make contact with the ground during a run or walk, your feet will bear two to three times your body weight per square inch; you must consider your body weight when shopping for shoes. Heavier runners/walkers (greater than 165 lbs) should look for:

■ A combination of cushioning, stability, and rearfoot control

■ A multi-density midsole with polyurethane and air or gel cushioning

■ A carbon rubber outsole

■ A straight or slightly curved shape

Conversely, lightweight runners/walkers should seek out lighter shoes with less cushioning and fewer motion control features.

Clue #4: Foot Type (Pronation and Supination)

Pronation means your feet roll excessively inward. *Supination* means your feet roll excessively outward. There is some natural pronation and supination of your feet during walking and running. These motions of the foot only become a problem if they are excessive. Knowing your foot type can make it easier to match your biomechanical needs to the characteristics of a shoe. To determine your foot type, wet your feet and step on a sheet of paper or dark pavement.

A Normal Foot:

Test results:	Shows an imprint with the toes and heels connected by a wide band
Shoe recommendations:	Nearly any shoe will work for normal feet. Moderate stability, arch-support, and cushion are appropriate.

A Flat Foot:

Test results:	Shows an imprint that looks like the whole sole of the foot, which indicates excessive pronation
Shoe recommendations:	Shoes with a firm midsole and motion-control features that reduce pronation

A High-Arched Foot:

Test results:	Shows an imprint with the toes and heel connected by a very narrow band, which indicates excessive supination
Shoe recommendations:	Shoes with plenty of flexibility and cushioning

Clue #5: Wear and Tear

If you exercise almost every day in one pair of shoes, they probably need to be replaced every three to six months. Excessive wear leads to a lack of support. It is helpful to have two pairs of shoes to alternate throughout the week. Monitor your shoes closely for signs of wear. Wear patterns can also indicate excessive pronation or supination of the foot, which can predispose you to injury if you are not wearing an appropriate shoe.

Signs of Normal Wear:

■ Scuffs on the outsole, over the middle area of the rearfoot, and middle area of toes and forefoot

■ The midsole, or area of shock absorption, begins to break down

■ The laces, toe-box, and other areas of the *upper* (the fabric above the sole) readily shows wear

Signs of Abnormal Wear:

■ Outside of the shoe begins to wear before any other part (indicates excessive supination)

■ Inner part of the shoe wears before any other part (indicates excessive pronation)

Clue #6: Surface Differences

The surface that you exercise on can make a difference in your performance and shoe wear.

Asphalt:

■ Good midsole shock absorbency is recommended

■ Good outsole durability is needed (outsole made of carbon rubber is more durable than other materials)

Track:

■ Less cushioning is necessary

■ More motion control is needed to help with the frequent turns on the track

Trails:

- Less cushioning is necessary
- More all-around support is recommended because trails often have varied terrain

Clue #7: Shoes to Choose Update

Watch for annual shoe surveys that appear in running and walking magazines and web sites. These surveys typically provide an expert analysis and ratings on the current shoes on the market.

What Safety Precautions Should Be Taken When Running and Walking in the Heat?

Summer brings many opportunities to participate in physical activities and sports. However, exercising in the summer heat and humidity can cause the body to work even harder than normal. Therefore, it is important to understand how to safely and effectively run and walk in the heat for proper body maintenance. The following tips can help keep your body comfortable, energetic, and safe.

Stay Well Hydrated

One key to surviving the summer sun is to stay hydrated. Thirst is not always a good indicator of hydration, so be sure to drink appropriate amounts of water on a regular basis throughout the day. Use the following guidelines to promote optimal hydration:

- Drink at least 8–12 cups of fluid each day (1 cup = 8 ounces). Consumption of water, milk, juice, coffee, tea, sports beverages, soda, and any other beverage counts toward your daily fluid goal.
- Drink two–three cups of fluid about two–three hours before exercising.
- Drink one cup of fluid 10–20 minutes before the workout.
- Drink at least one cup of fluid every 10–20 minutes during exercise.
- After exercise, a general rule is to consume two–three cups for every pound of body weight lost during exercise.
- 100% fruit/vegetable juice and milk are excellent options for fluids after exercise; juice replaces lost fluids, electrolytes, and carbohydrates, while milk provides a perfect balance of carbohydrate and protein.

Proper Clothing

In warm weather, ideal clothing consists of material that allows for the evaporation of sweat and moisture from the skin. Evaporation and the transfer of moisture keep the body cool and prevent chafing. Clothing made from rubber or plastic prevents evaporative cooling and should *never* be worn in warm weather conditions. Cotton clothing is also not a good choice of fabric because cotton absorbs moisture and keeps the skin wet. Additional guidelines to follow when choosing warm weather clothes include the following:

- Warm weather clothing should be loose fitting to permit the free circulation of air between the skin and the environment, thereby promoting sweat evaporation from the skin.
- Wear light-colored clothing to better reflect the sun's rays away from the body.
- Make sure clothing is lightweight and wicks moisture away from the skin. Materials such as polypropylene wick moisture away from the body and are excellent choices. Remember—no cotton!

Prevention Is Key

The most effective way to control heat-related problems is to prevent them. The first key to preventing heat-related problems is to properly acclimate yourself to the heat. Train slowly, gradually increasing your time outdoors. It takes 7–14 days to become acclimated to the heat. The time of day is also an important factor when exercising. Try to avoid exercising between 10 a.m. and 3 p.m., which are often the hottest times of the day. Refer to the Apparent Temperature Chart shown in Figure 4.1 for precautions when exercising in the heat.

HEAT-RELATED ILLNESSES

Runners and walkers are more susceptible to heat illnesses than sedentary individuals. However, everyone needs to take special precautions during summer training sessions. The heat and humidity frequently experienced during summer months can be downright dangerous. Heat and humidity cause the body to work harder. If the humidity is very high, the body cannot cool itself efficiently because water cannot evaporate from the skin. If an individual has a prolonged exposure to summer conditions and becomes dehydrated, heat illnesses can occur. If these conditions are left untreated, the situation can become fatal. It is critical that everyone is familiar with the signs, symptoms, and treatment for heat exhaustion and heat stroke.

Symptoms of Heat Exhaustion:

- Progressive weakness, reduced appetite
- Moist, clammy skin

continues

- Pulse rapid but weak
- Common for fainting to occur

Treatment of Heat Exhaustion:

- Remove as much clothing as possible
- Apply ice packs on pressure points, especially near the carotid artery in the neck and the femoral artery near the top of the thigh/groin area
- Drink cool water
- Remove the runner/walker from heat or direct sun for the rest of the day
- If the runner/walker does not feel better shortly, take him/her to a hospital

Symptoms of Heat Stroke:

- Dizziness, weakness, and confusion
- May be or become unconscious
- High temperature, 105 degrees is not uncommon
- Skin is flushed, hot, and dry

Treatment of Heat Stroke:

- Get the runner/walker to a doctor
- Follow first aid for heat exhaustion until the person can be admitted to a hospital.

FIGURE 4.1

Decrease outdoor exercise duration and intensity when conditions are within the "Caution" or "Extreme Caution" ranges. Exercise indoors in a cool, climate-controlled environment when outdoor conditions are in the "Danger" or "Extreme Danger" ranges.

Apparent Temperature Chart

Air Temperature (°F)	0	5	10	15	20	25	30	35	40	45	50	55	60	65	70	75	80	85	90	95	100
120	108	112	117	124	131	135															
115	104	107	110	116	120	128	138														
110	99	102	105	108	112	117	123	130	139												
105	95	98	100	102	105	108	113	117	122	130	140	155									
100	91	93	95	97	98	102	104	107	110	115	120	126	132	138							
95	86	88	89	91	93	95	98	100	104	106	109	113	119	124	130	136	142	147	153	155	
90	82	84	85	86	87	88	90	91	92	95	97	98	100	103	106	110	114	117	121	125	130
85	77	78	80	81	82	83	84	85	86	87	87	89	90	92	94	96	97	100	102	105	108
80	73	74	75	76	77	78	78	79	79	80	81	82	83	84	85	86	87	88	88	90	92
75	69	70	70	71	71	72	73	74	74	75	75	76	76	76	77	77	77	78	78	79	80
70	65	65	66	66	67	67	68	68	68	68	69	69	70	70	70	71	71	72	72	73	73

Relative Humidity (%)

Caution: Fatigue possible with prolonged exposure and physical activity (80° to 89°F).

Extreme Caution: Sunstroke, Heat Cramps, or Heat Exhaustion possible with prolonged exposure and physical activity (90° to 104°F).

Danger: Sunstroke, Heat Cramps, or Heat Exhaustion likely; Heatstroke possible with prolonged exposure and physical activity (105° to 129°F).

Extreme Danger: Heatstroke or Sunstroke imminent (130°F or more).

Watch weather conditions closely and use common sense when exercising in the heat. Consult the Apparent Temperature Chart before exercising and practice heat illness prevention techniques.

What Safety Precautions Should Be Taken When Running and Walking in the Cold?

Just as exercising in the warm weather can be dangerous, the same applies to exercising in the cold. The human body possesses a lesser capacity for adaptation to prolonged cold exposure than to long-term exposure to heat. As a result, there are several safety considerations for effectively preparing the body to exercise in the cold.

Stay Well Hydrated

To survive the cold, proper hydration is of utmost importance. Even though you might not notice it as much as during the summer months, you can lose a significant amount of body fluid through sweat even in cold temperatures. Refer to the hydration guidelines presented in the "What Safety Precautions Should Be Taken When Running and Walking in the Heat?" section earlier in this chapter for the appropriate quantities and timing of fluids consumption.

Proper Clothing

The predominant concern when faced with exercising in cold environments is to properly cover exposed areas of skin. If there is one key to properly clothing yourself, it is to remember to cover your head during exercise. A person's head can lose up to one half the body's total heat production at 39°F when not covered. Although there are many options for proper clothing, the ideal cold weather garment is impermeable to air movement, but permits the escape of water vapor from the skin when sweating occurs. When shopping for clothing and dressing for a cold-weather walk or run, keep in mind the following:

- The clothing layer closest to the skin must be effective in taking moisture away from the body.
- After this first layer add an insulating layer to keep the body from losing warmth.
- Synthetics, such as polypropylene, work best for allowing the garment to dry quickly, keeping you warm and comfortable.

Be Aware of the Wind Chill

One problem in evaluating the actual temperature in the environment is that a normal temperature reading is not always a valid indication of coldness. The factor that must also be analyzed is that of wind velocity. Wind velocity combined with air temperature produces a reading referred to as *wind chill*. Wind chill provides a more accurate estimation of the severity of weather conditions. For example, an air temperature of 30°F is equivalent to a wind chill reading of 0°F when the wind speed is 25 mph. The Wind Chill Chart shown in Figure 4.2 can be used to safely analyze the actual temperature readings before your next cold weather exercise session.

caution

Avoid outdoor exercise or limit exposure to less than the stated time for frostbite to occur as temperatures dip below zero with even mild winds.

SLOW

FIGURE 4.2

Frostbite can occur rapidly when temperatures drop and wind speeds increase. Limit outdoor activities as temperatures approach 0–10 degrees.

Frostbite Times

□ 30 minutes

□ 10 minutes

■ 5 minutes

Wind Chill Chart

Wind (mph)	Temperature (°F)								
Calm	40	30	20	10	0	-10	-20	-30	-40
5	36	25	13	1	-11	-22	-34	-46	-57
10	34	21	9	-4	-16	-28	-41	-53	-66
15	32	19	6	-7	-19	-32	-45	-58	-71
20	30	17	4	-9	-22	-35	-48	-61	-74
25	29	16	3	-11	-24	-37	-51	-64	-78
30	28	15	1	-12	-26	-39	-53	-67	-80
35	28	14	0	-14	-27	-41	-55	-69	-82
40	27	13	-1	-15	-29	-43	-57	-71	-84
45	26	12	-2	-16	-30	-44	-58	-72	-86
50	26	12	-3	-17	-31	-45	-60	-74	-88
55	25	11	-3	-18	-32	-46	-61	-75	-89
60	25	10	-4	-19	-33	-48	-62	-76	-91

What Is the Key to Dressing for Success?

The previous section discussed the types of fabrics to choose for running and walking in a wide range of temperatures. However, knowing only the type of fabric to wear does not answer all the questions. Should you wear a short sleeve or long sleeve? Shorts or pants? A jacket or a vest? Sometimes the answer is obvious and other times it is not. Don't forget that you warm up once you start running and walking. You should feel slightly chilled when you walk out the front door in cool weather; if you feel comfortable, you are overdressed. Table 4.1 provides some ideas on clothing to wear, whatever the weather.

note

Running or walking automatically raises your body temperature. It will feel about 20 degrees warmer than the actual temperature outdoors while running or walking, so you need to dress accordingly. You should feel a slight chill when you step outdoors. If you feel comfortable before beginning your walk or run, you have over-dressed.

Table 4.1   Dressing for Success: How to Be Comfortable, Whatever the Weather

Weather	Temperature Ranges	Clothing Choices
Hot	70°F and higher	Tank-singlet, shorts
Warm	50°F to 69°F	Short sleeve T-shirt, shorts
Cool	30°F to 49°F	Comfortable windpants, long sleeve T-shirt and light-weight jacket if needed
Cold	29°F and below	Layer running tights, long sleeve shirts, light-weight jacket; protect head, ears and hands with hats, ear warmers, and gloves
Warm/Rain	50°F to 69°F	Wear a cap and reflective gear for visibility, avoid 100% cotton as it absorbs water and becomes heavy
Cool/Rain	30°F to 49°F	Cap, water repellent, and reflective jacket and pants

RUNNING AND WALKING TRAINING GADGETS—REFLECTIVE GEAR AND IDENTIFICATION

Safety while walking and running outdoors is of utmost importance. Wear reflective gear so automobiles, bikes, and other walkers/runners can see you even at night. Carrying identification is critical if an accident does occur and you need medical attention. The following products are examples of what is on the market to keep you "illuminated" and prepared. All descriptions taken directly from the products' websites.

- *Road ID BrightGear™ Wrist* (www.roadid.com)—This bright neon yellow wristband is comfortable and fully adjustable. Highly visible in the dark, it will keep you safe from traffic and other exercisers.

- *Petzl Tikka Plus Headlamp* (www.petzl.com)—For both runners and walkers, this comfortable and fully adjustable headband holds a lamp for lighting your way. The lamp has three brightness settings that will provide light for up to 150 hours and close to 400 hours on the blinking mode.

- *Sugoi MicroFine Reflective Cap* (www.sugoi.ca)—This water-resistant and breathable cap is trimmed with reflective binding for visibility in the dark.

- *New Balance® Tepid Training Vest* (www.newbalance.com)—This lightweight vest is perfect for spring and fall walks and runs. Reflective piping runs along the vest for visibility in the rain or at night.

- *Adidas® Adistar Rain Jacket* (www.adidas.com)—This breathable jacket is perfect for cool, rainy days. Reflective detailing on the front, arms, and back provides illumination and safety in low-light and dark conditions.

- *Nathan & Co. Reflective Safety Vest* (www.roadrunnersports.com)—An absolute essential for any walker or runner, this lightweight vest can be placed over any type of apparel, ranging from summer to winter gear. The bright reflective bands run horizontally and vertically allowing drivers to see you up to 1,200 feet away. One size fits all.

- *RRS Reflective Kit* (www.roadrunnersports.com)—For the full spectrum of reflective materials/gear, this kit provides stick-on reflective strips and dots, a clip-on reflective yield symbol, and a safety band that reflects and flashes at the same time for maximum visibility.

- *Road ID Shoe ID* (www.roadid.com)—The Shoe ID consists of a stainless steel metal plate engraved with up to six lines of text (such as name, phone number, address, and critical medical information). The plate is attached to a small, reflective, Velcro strap that is attached to the laces of your walking or running shoes.

What Is the Best Way to Deal with Dog Encounters While Walking and Running?

Dogs are pets, so that means they must all be nice and friendly, right? Wrong. All of us have probably come across at least one dog while on a path, trail, or in our neighborhoods. Some dogs ignore our presence, whereas others can scare the pants off us with their charges, mean looks, and growls. Dogs, whether domesticated or not, still have the instinct to be territorial often paired with a predatory predisposition. In certain circumstances, dogs can cause severe injury or death to people. When running and walking outdoors, you need to be prepared to act accordingly when you sight a dog to stay healthy and unharmed.

before you head out the door

Make sure you have some form of identification with you at all times. Remember to put on reflective gear if it is dark outside or will become dark before the end of your walk or run.

Understanding "Dog Talk"

To best protect yourself, it is important to understand canine behavior and how to act in response. According to the Humane Society of the United States:

- Learn how to read a dog's body language and know when to keep away. A frightened animal holds its ears down, tucks its tail under its body, and may shake, growl, or back away. Trying to befriend it invites an attack.

- Stay clear of a dog that is angry or aggressively protecting its territory: Ears are up and forward; eyes look directly at you; tail is up and may be wagging slowly; hair may be standing up on the neck, back, and tail; and the dog is likely to be barking or growling with teeth exposed.

- If you are approached by an aggressive dog, do not run. Running only stimulates the dog to increase its aggression. The best defense is to freeze. Act like a tree: Stand perfectly still with hands in fists held close to the body, don't yell or say anything, and *don't* look at the animal. Dogs interpret direct eye contact as a threat or challenge.

- If a dog knocks you down, act like a rock: Roll into a fetal position with knees up, elbows tucked in, and hands in fists held against your ears.

- If you are charged by a dog, don't yell or scream, but immediately offer an article of clothing, gym bag, purse, or other item for the animal to tug on.

■ If a dog should grab your arm or leg, push into its mouth as hard as you can. It will make the dog feel it is losing control and it will let go and run. This will also keep your flesh from tearing on the dog's teeth as you push away.

OTHER HELPFUL SAFETY HINTS

The following are some additional ways you can keep safe when you run or walk:

■ Choose a running or walking route that is well lit.

■ Find friends to train with; running/walking in groups is safer than alone.

■ Know where emergency phones or businesses are located along your chosen route in case of an emergency. Many water bottle waist belts will also have a pouch for a cell phone.

■ Notify a friend or family member when you are heading out for a walk or run by yourself, including your planned route and distance.

■ Carry emergency information with you at all times.

■ Walk and run on even surfaces to avoid injuring yourself while on the course, potentially far away from your car, home, or other exercisers.

THE ABSOLUTE MINIMUM

■ Take time to find the best fitting shoes for your feet. Shop at a reputable athletic, running, or walking store with trained, experienced professionals on staff.

■ Stay well hydrated during the hot days of summer as well as the frigid days of winter.

■ Purchase and wear running and walking gear made from wicking fabrics that will keep you dry and comfortable.

■ Wear reflective gear.

■ Consult temperature charts to determine whether you need to make modifications to your workout (such as shortened distance, extra fluids, additional clothing, and so on).

■ Learn how to interpret the actions of dogs and respond accordingly during a walk or run.

■ Be serious about safety!

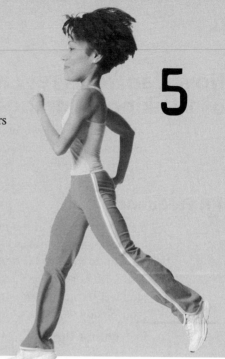

IN THIS CHAPTER

- Training errors that lead to injuries
- Common injuries of runners and walkers
- Prevention tips for common injuries
- Immediate first aid for injuries
- Preventing overtraining

5

INJURY PREVENTION AND TREATMENT

Running and walking should not hurt.

The phrase "no pain, no gain" is obsolete. Running and walking should be a fun, relaxing form of exercise—it should not be painful and miserable. Running and walking should challenge your body to improve and adapt, but it should not cause pain and discomfort, especially if it lasts for hours or days after a running or walking session. This chapter will teach you to be aware of the warning signs that indicate first aid or a trip to the doctor is needed, and more importantly, how you can prevent aches and pains from ever occurring!

How Can You Prevent the 13 Common Causes of Walking/Running-Related Injuries?

Injuries happen. However, they are not inevitable. You can dramatically decrease your risk for any exercise-related injury by being aware of the common causes for injuries and how to prevent them through smart training.

#1: Frequency

A sudden increase in the number of times per week you exercise can result in an injury. If you are walking two times a week and you wish to do more, gradually work up to three walks a week, and then four walks, and then five walks, as you desire. Do not suddenly increase by two or three sessions per week. Although you may feel strong at the time, a sudden progression can add up to an injury down the road. Steady as you go!

Prevention tips:

- Progress gradually.
- Increase exercise frequency by no more than one day per week.
- Always take at least one day off each week for rest and recovery.

#2: Intensity

The periods before and after an exercise session are critical times for preventing unnecessary pain and injury. The purpose of a warm-up is to prepare your body, especially your cardiorespiratory and musculoskeletal systems, for activity. Warming up allows your body temperature to increase slightly, loosens up your joints and muscles, allows your heart and lungs to efficiently operate, reduces your risk of injury, and mentally helps prepare you for the workout. The key to a proper warm-up is to begin slowly and gradually increase the intensity. The warm-up movements should be a slow version of the activity you are about to do—basically slow walking or jogging. You should always end an exercise session with 5–10 minutes of cool-down to allow your body to recover. This allows your heart rate, blood pressure, and body temperature to gradually return to a pre-exercise condition. Never stop exercising abruptly. Instead, continue moving at a slower pace until your body stops sweating.

Prevention tips:

- Warm up for 5–10 minutes before a walk or run during which the intensity should be 40%–60% of your maximum heart rate.
- Cool down for 5–10 minutes after a walk or run and then stretch.

#3: Progression of Exercise Intensity

If you are comfortable exercising at 50%–65% of your target heart rate range and feel ready to increase the effort, exercise at a slightly higher intensity level (70%–75%) for a portion of your exercise session, but not all of it. Then for future exercise sessions, increase the number of minutes you exercise at the higher intensity until you can comfortably exercise at that level for a full workout. Too much intensity too soon will lead to discomfort, nausea, and undue fatigue. Many people report they dropped out of a running or walking program because it did not feel good. Don't let this happen to you. It's your body and you are in control of your exercise level. Make exercise enjoyable and comfortable by walking and running at a moderate intensity level and gradually progressing over time.

Prevention tip:

■ Progress exercise intensity gradually, in small segments over several weeks.

#4: Duration

As with frequency and intensity, a safe and effective running/walking program will gradually increase the total number of minutes you exercise over time. A good rule of thumb is to increase your cardiorespiratory exercise time by no more than 5%–10% a week. Even if you are excited about exercise, avoid walking or running too much too soon. An injury may cause you to be sidelined during time you could have been steadily progressing. Be aware that the greatest number of injuries occur at the end of a hard day of activity or an extended exercise session.

Prevention tips:

■ Do not increase mileage or exercise time by more than 5%–10% per week.

■ Do not increase mileage or exercise time every week; predetermine recovery weeks when mileage or exercise time will be maintained or decreased.

note

The 5%–10% rule is essential to preventing injuries while training for a 5K, 10K, or half-marathon. The protocols in this book have built in the 5%–10% rule; do not allow yourself to be tempted to walk or run more than planned.

#5: Speed

If you are interested in improving your speed, do so in steady, progressive bouts. Because you are a beginner, you should not attempt any type of speed work until after 12–16 weeks of easy running/walking. Then, you can add one session per week of 4–6 gradual accelerations lasting 60 seconds and ending with the last 15 seconds slightly faster than 5K, 10K, or half-marathon goal pace. Run or walk easy for two minutes between each acceleration. Do this for six weeks, adding one acceleration per week. Do not do more than two faster speed-work sessions per week. Let your body strengthen and adapt gradually to the demands you place on it.

Prevention tips:

- If you are just trying to finish a 5K, 10K, or half-marathon, train at half-marathon goal pace or slower. Do not attempt speed work.
- Do not attempt faster-paced training until after 12–16 weeks of easy consistent training.
- Weekly training volume of faster-paced training should not exceed 20%–25% of total weekly mileage.

#6: Stretching

Stretching limbers up tight muscles and reduces your risk for sprains and tears. Concentrate on stretching the muscles you will be using during walking and running. Stretching after exercise helps minimize muscle soreness. A quality exercise program of any type should include stretches.

Prevention tips:

- Spend at least 10–20 minutes total each day stretching.
- Stretch after warm-up and after cool-down.
- Static stretching is best for increasing flexibility and preventing injuries.
- See Chapter 7, "Warm-Up/Cool-Down and Flexibility Exercises," for details and instructions on specific stretches for walkers and runners.

#7: Body Fat Percentage

The more you weigh the greater amount of shock and stress your body sustains in activities such as running and high-impact aerobics. However, a body heavy with muscle is stronger than a body heavy with fat. If you are "overfat," (body fat percentage of greater than 20% for men and 25% for women) walking or non-weight bearing activities such as bicycling, swimming, or other water exercises are recommended to reduce the risk of injury while you are getting in shape. After you have

note

Your body fat percentage can be determined through a body composition assessment. The results of this test will reveal your current amount of lean weight and fat weight. The ratio of your fat weight to your total weight provides your body fat percentage.

lowered your body fat percentage into a healthy range, you can progress to running, if desired.

Prevention tips:

- Schedule an appointment with an exercise specialist to determine your body composition.

- Engage in 30–60 minutes of physical activity on most days of the week.

- Incorporate non-weight bearing activities into your training program.

- Focus on a balanced, varied diet; see a registered dietitian to answer your questions and help you establish a plan.

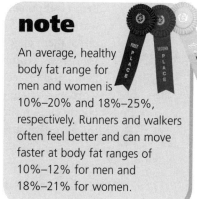

note

An average, healthy body fat range for men and women is 10%–20% and 18%–25%, respectively. Runners and walkers often feel better and can move faster at body fat ranges of 10%–12% for men and 18%–21% for women.

HOW CAN YOU FIND AN EXERCISE SPECIALIST OR REGISTERED DIETITIAN IN YOUR AREA?

Exercise specialists are typically employed in fitness centers, corporate health sites, medical facilities, and some health-related non-profit organizations. Ask for an exercise specialist who has an exercise science degree from an accredited college or university and who is certified by the American College of Sports Medicine or the National Strength and Conditioning Association. Dietitians are typically employed in medical facilities, some fitness centers and health-related non-profit organizations, or in private practice. The American Dietetics Association has an online service to locate dietitians in your area who specifically work with runners, walkers, and other sports-minded individuals. Go to www.eatright.org and click on "Find a Nutrition Professional" to locate a certified dietitian in your area.

#8: Exercising Surfaces

Concrete, tile, wood, carpet, asphalt, and grass can cause injuries from exercising on hard, slippery, uneven surfaces or rough terrain.

Prevention tip:

- Search for even, soft surfaces for running and walking training sessions.

#9: Choosing a Shoe

Not choosing the proper footwear is one of the most common mistakes people make when beginning a walking or running program. If your exercise shoes are not designed for the activity for which you are using them, you may not be getting the protection you need. The cushioning used to absorb exercise impact, and the stabilizing components used to control the foot and ankle from excessive inward and outward roll, are placed differently in each athletic shoe. Although the shoe design may make them effective for one sport, it does not mean they are appropriate for all sports. For example, a basketball shoe is designed for lateral movements, thus stabilizing and protecting the ankles. However, they are not designed for repetitive forward movement and impact, so they are not appropriate for running or walking. Poorly chosen shoes not only increase the risk for foot and ankle injuries, but also the excessive stress on your feet can translate into hip, knee, or back problems.

Shoes must also match your specific body mechanics (how you move). Your arch height, heel strike, foot roll, and body weight play a role in determining which shoes are best designed for you. Choose walking and running shoes from a quality athletic shoe store where the salespeople ask to see you walk, run, or jump in the shoes. By analyzing your movement, they can determine which shoes are the best for you. Structural differences such as curvature of the spine, unequal leg length, bowlegs, or knock-knees can be accommodated by wearing proper shoes or shoe orthotics from a sports medicine specialist or podiatrist.

Ideally, you should have two pairs of walking/running shoes and wear them on alternate days. Wearing old worn shoes during a walk or run session can open up the door for injury.

Prevention tips:

- Consult a knowledgeable salesperson at a reputable athletic store for advice on which shoe is best for you.
- Monitor your shoes for wear and tear indicating the need for a new pair.
- As a general rule, purchase new running/walking shoes every 300–500 miles.

before you head out the door

Make sure you are wearing the appropriate shoes for walking and running, and then complete the designated walking or running mileage for the day—don't be tempted to go further.

#10: Safety Devices

Various pieces of equipment are needed to protect your body during running, walking, and cross training sessions. Safety gear may feel awkward or look "funny," but these inconveniences are far outweighed by the reduced risk of injury.

Prevention tips:

- ▓ Helmets, goggles, sunglasses, mitts, braces, and pads are a few of the safety devices available for an active person.

- ▓ For skin protection and safety, apply plenty of sunscreen of SPF (Sun Protection Factor) 15 frequently.

- ▓ Wear a reflective vest when training outdoors at night.

- ▓ Use Vaseline®, BodyGlide® or other lubricating agents on areas of the body that are easily irritated to prevent chafing.

RUNNING AND WALKING TRAINING GADGETS—BODYGLIDE

Chafing can range from a mild irritation to pure agony. Chafing occurs when clothing, body parts, or other running/walking accessories rub an area of the body until it becomes red, raw, and inflamed. If the chafing is excessive, it can lead to blisters or bloody cuts. I highly recommend buying this product or one similar to it, and use it liberally. You will know where it should go after your first couple of walks/runs; however the typical "hot spots" are under the arms, in the groin area, and the nipples for men. It is also great for preventing blisters on your feet and in between your toes! Description taken directly from product website.

Made from plant-derived waxes, BODYGLIDE® (www.sternoff.com) is a non-greasy lubricant that guards skin from the friction that causes chafing and blisters. It is water-resistant, uniquely allowing your skin to breathe while still providing lubrication. BODYGLIDE comes in a twist-up tube, gliding on your body without a mess.

#11: Orthopedic Limitations

If you have an orthopedic limitation such as arthritis or back, knee, ankle, or shoulder problems, you can still exercise but you may need to make some modifications in the frequency, duration, or type of exercise. Ignoring physical limitations can result in overstressing the area, ultimately leading to injury. A fitness screening or a visit with a sports medicine specialist can help you identify orthopedic limitations that exist, as well as the associated exercise modifications that are necessary to remain healthy.

Prevention tip:

- ▓ Consult an exercise specialist or sports medicine doctor about appropriate exercise modifications.

#12: Inadequate Leadership/Poor Program Design

Exercise injuries may also stem from inadequate leadership or poor program design. Knowledgeable exercise leaders should have university degrees in exercise physiology, exercise science, or physical education, and hold certification by organizations such as the American College of Sports Medicine (ACSM), National Strength and Conditioning Association (NSCA), or other recognized certifying bodies. Group fitness instructors also should be certified by credible associations such as ACSM, the International Association of Fitness Professionals (IDEA), the American Council on Exercise (ACE), or the Aerobic and Fitness Association of America (AFAA).

Prevention tips:

- Closely follow the schedule in this book that is appropriate for you; all of the protocols have been created by experienced, knowledgeable, certified staff members from the National Institute for Fitness and Sport (NIFS) in Indianapolis.
- NIFS staff members are degreed, certified individuals; please ask us your questions! We can be reached at 317.274.3432 or www.nifs.org.
- Set realistic goals.

#13: Returning from an Injury

If an injury has caused you to miss your typical running and walking sessions for an extended period of time (two weeks or more), you must return slowly and easily. The first few weeks back are crucial in preventing future injuries in the same area. Exercising recovering areas too hard makes you more susceptible to re-injury.

Prevention tips:

- Return to walking and running gradually.
- Follow the previously discussed rules for increasing the frequency, intensity, and duration of your training.
- Listen to your body; modify your training schedule accordingly.

caution

Do *not* "walk/run through" an injury. If you begin to feel aches and pains that linger for days or weeks, do not ignore the symptoms. Too many walkers and runners push past the early signs of an injury, which can lead to more serious complications and time off of training down the road.

What Are Some of the Common Walking and Running Injuries?

As mentioned earlier, injuries can happen. It is important to be aware of the signs and symptoms of commonly diagnosed injuries in order to recognize the problem and know when to seek medical attention. The sooner you implement treatment strategies, the more rapidly you will recover and be able to return to walking and running. See Table 5.1 for some of the more commonly diagnosed injuries experienced by runners and walkers.

Table 5.1 Commonly Diagnosed Injuries for Runner and Walkers

Injury	Symptoms	Prevention	Treatment
Blisters	Irritated area of skin that is filled with fluid or blood.	Purchase shoes specific to the needs of your feet and break in new shoes gradually.	Lubricate the area or wear two pairs of socks to decrease friction; do not puncture the blister because this invites infection.
Shin splints	Pain in the lower leg, specifically on the anterior/medial side (front/inside).	Strengthen and stretch the muscles in the front and back of the lower leg; wear well-fitting shoes.	Cross train with non-impact exercises; ice the affected area several times a day; return to running and walking slowly after pain subsides.
Muscle strains	Pain directly over the injured area of the muscle; stiffness or tightness when the muscle is worked or stretched.	Warm up thoroughly before walking and running; stretch for 10–20 minutes after a walk or run.	Use the R.I.C.E. principle: Rest, Ice, Compression, and Elevation; stretch lightly but be careful not to overstretch to the point of pain; cross train to use other muscle groups.
Ligament sprains	Instability around a joint; pain in a specific area of the joint; swelling and bruising typically occur.	Perform resistance-training exercises regularly to strengthen muscles and ligaments; wear appropriate shoes.	See your physician to determine the severity of the injury; use the R.I.C.E. principle; perform exercises that do not involve the injured area of the body.

Table 5.1 (continued)

Injury	Symptoms	Prevention	Treatment
Plantar fasciitis	Pain on the bottom of the foot, from mid-sole to near the heel (but not directly on the heel). Pain is at its worst in the morning.	Wear appropriate shoes; stretch the muscles of the lower leg and the plantar fascia (bottom of foot).	Cross train with non-weight bearing exercises; ice the affected area several times a day; wear supportive shoes throughout the day; orthotics may be indicated.
Stress fractures	Gradual onset of pain in a specific bony area, such as the foot or leg.	Increase training duration, frequency, and intensity appropriately; buy new shoes every 300–500 miles; return from an injury gradually.	Cross train using non-weight bearing modes of exercise; use the R.I.C.E. principle after exercising; see your physician for further instructions based on the severity of the injury.
Neuromas	Pain in the ball of the foot or in between the toes; a tingling, radiating sensation is common.	Wear appropriately fitting shoes (problem often caused by shoes that squeeze or restrict the forefoot/toes).	Use the R.I.C.E. principle after exercise; purchase different work and/or exercise shoes; cross train using non-weight bearing modes of exercise.

If You Do Get Injured, What Should You Do?

Many injuries can be prevented by proper conditioning and stretching after activity. However, when an injury does occur, the manner in which it is handled can make a difference in the length of recovery time needed. Sudden swelling will occur with an injury due to bleeding or inflammation of the injured area. The acronym R.I.C.E. (Rest, Ice, Compression, and Elevation) can help you remember how to treat injuries to reduce swelling in the area, thus speeding recovery time.

R.I.C.E. can be used for short-term treatment of sprains, strains, fractures, or joint injuries. Immediate treatment with R.I.C.E. is important because swelling can start within 10 seconds after an injury. Keep in mind that R.I.C.E. is not a substitute for medical attention; if pain and swelling persist, additional treatments may be indicated.

R = Rest

As soon as you realize that an injury has taken place, stop activity immediately; continuing to exercise may cause further damage. Resting the injured area is critical for proper healing. However, a modified exercise program can be continued as long as it is not painful to the injured area.

- Using crutches for injuries of the foot, ankle, knee, and leg is recommended to keep the weight off the injured area.

- Splints are recommended for injuries to the hand, wrist, elbow, and arm to keep the area immobilized.

note

Do not try to self-diagnose the injuries discussed in Table 5.1. If you feel pain, see your physician to confirm a diagnosis, determine the severity of the injury, discuss various treatment options, and implement any necessary adjustments to your training program.

I = Ice

Swelling is a natural, protective reaction that cushions and splints an injury preventing motion. However, the excess fluid pressing on the nerves in the injured area causes pain. Ice reduces swelling, muscle spasms, and pain by constricting blood vessels, which decreases blood flow to the injured area. Ice also decreases the pooling of blood within the injured tissues, which results in faster healing.

- Cover the entire injury when applying ice.

- For small body parts, immerse the injured area in a cup (for fingers) or bucket (for ankles) of ice water; use ice packs for larger areas (such as your knee).

- Apply ice for 20–30 minutes, for the first 48–72 hours, three to four times a day.

C = Compression

Compressing the injured area decreases the swelling by limiting blood and plasma flow.

- Apply compression by wrapping the injury with an elastic wrap whenever possible.

- Wet the bandage before wrapping to facilitate the transfer of coolness from the ice to the injury.

- Begin wrapping below the injured area and move in a circular motion toward the center of the body.

- Be sure that the wrap is not pulled too tight that it restricts or occludes circulation.

- Apply ice after the compression wrap is completed.

E = Elevation

Elevate the injured area above the level of the heart to allow gravity to help drain excess fluid and further decrease swelling in the area.

- Elevate after the wet bandage and ice packs are applied during compression.

- Elevate a lower extremity overnight by placing a pillow underneath the mattress.

caution

Pain, numbness, cramping, and blue or dusky colored nails are all signs of blood deprivation. Remove compression bandage immediately if any of these symptoms occur. When the symptoms are gone, rewrap the area less tightly.

When to See a Physician

If swelling and pain persist after three days, consult with your physician. An X-ray may be needed to rule out the possibility of a fracture.

Is More Training Always Better?

Many times when individuals are involved in an exercise program they establish goals and develop a strong motivation to attain those goals. Mistakenly, some individuals may begin to think, "The more I train, the better my performance." Unfortunately, this theory can lead to *overtraining*. Overtraining means that you have stressed your body past its limits, resulting in a state of catabolism (breakdown) which overrides the body's ability to adapt and repair (anabolism). Table 5.2 lists the physiological, psychological, and performance effects of overtraining.

note

Submaximal heart rates are any heart rates below your predicted maximum (your age subtracted from 220). If you are overtrained, you will notice that your heart rate during exercise is higher than in weeks prior while performing the same activity, at the same intensity.

Table 5.2   The Damaging Effects of Overtraining

Physiological	Psychological	Performance
Excessive weight loss	Depression	Early onset of fatigue
Excessive loss of body fat	Loss of appetite	Decreased aerobic capacity
Increased resting heart rate	Irritability	
Decreased muscular strength	Loss of motivation	Poor race performance
Increased submaximal heart rate	Loss of enthusiasm	Inability to complete workouts
Inability to complete workouts	Loss of competitive drive	
Chronic muscle soreness		Delayed recovery
Fatigue		
Increased incidence of injury		
Depressed immune system		
Constipation or diarrhea		
Absence of menstruation		
Frequent minor infections/colds		
Insomnia		

Misconceptions/Attitudes That Lead to Overtraining

Overtraining often can occur when individuals have an inappropriate perspective of proper training. It is essential for you to know your limits and abilities. The following are myths, misconceptions, or attitudes about exercise that can lead to overtraining:

- ▪ *The more, the better.* More is not always better. Follow a conservative plan and stick with it.

- ▪ *Failure to heed your body's warning signs.* If you begin to feel unusually fatigued or sore, take a couple extra days off from walking/running to allow your body to rest and recover. Don't forget that work, family, and other life responsibilities can cause fatigue as well as training—you may need to cut back on other commitments to make time for proper training and rest.

- ▪ *No pain, no gain.* Walking and running should not be painful. Pain is a sign that something is not quite right.

- ▪ *Lack of sufficient/quality recovery.* Rest days are important. Do not skip a rest day to fit in more walking, running, or other modes of exercise. Take advantage of these days to allow your body to be refreshed and renewed for your next workout. It is actually during your time off from training that your body adapts and becomes stronger.

- *"If she does 70 miles per week then I should too."* Do not compare yourself to others. Choose a plan that works for you and stick with it.

- *Too much, too fast.* Slow and steady like the tortoise wins the race; ease into running and walking and enjoy the process.

- *Too much at too high of an intensity.* Keep the intensity of your walks and runs moderate for several months before attempting to increase the intensity and/or incorporate any type of speed work.

- *"My performance will suffer if I take a day off."* It can't be said enough: Honor your days off and allow your body to repair and replenish. And do not underestimate the power of sleep!

Smart Nutrition

Proper nutrition is essential for the body to function properly. Replenishing the body with nutrients immediately after walking and running sessions will allow for improved performance and recovery, as well as the prevention of overtraining.

- Eat a well-balanced meal as soon as possible after a walk or run; the meal should consist of both carbohydrates (such as whole grains, fruits, and vegetables) and protein (such as meat, dairy, or meat/dairy alternatives).

- Drink to replenish your sweat losses after walking or running; for every pound that you lose, drink two to three cups of fluid. Fluids can be obtained by consuming 100% fruit or vegetables juices, milk, or water.

Smart Training

Smart training practices can prevent overtraining. To gain the most from your workout, improve your performance, and prevent overtraining, implement the following training guidelines:

- *Listen to your body!* Listen to your body and complete the workload it can handle, as well as what is optimal for your 5K, 10K, or half-marathon goals.

- Stretch at least 10–20 minutes after each workout.

- Include one cross training day each week. Choose an exercise that is different from walking and running to utilize a variety of muscle groups throughout the body.

- Avoid training at the same intensity each workout. Vary intensity from easy (most days) to moderate-hard (1–2 days/week, after several months of training).

- Do not increase weekly mileage by more than 5%–10%; in some cases, you may want to wait two to three weeks before increasing your mileage again.

- Plan your recovery as well as you plan your training.

- Plan to taper 5–10 days before your planned 5K, 10K, or half-marathon by reducing your weekly mileage by up to 50%; a taper has already been incorporated into all of the training protocols in this book.

- Keep a training log to review previous workouts, performances, and physical and psychological status.

THE ABSOLUTE MINIMUM

- Avoid the common training errors that can potentially lead to injury.

- Implement the R.I.C.E. principle immediately following an injury.

- Seek medical attention for any walking- or running-related pain that persists for more than three days.

- Follow your chosen walking or running 5K, 10K, or half-marathon protocol and the associated training guidelines to avoid overtraining.

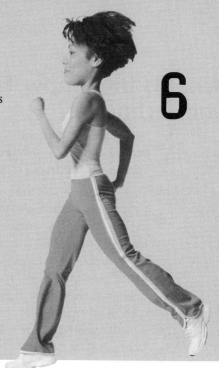

6

PROPER WALKING AND RUNNING FORM

Improve the way you move for "easy," pain-free walking and running.

Do you ever wonder why some people make walking and running look so easy and effortless? Have you wished that you could walk or run similarly? You can! By focusing on some basic guidelines for improving fitness walking, racewalking, and running form, you can begin to experience "easy" walking and running. Improving the way you move also decreases the risk of developing an athletic-related injury, which will keep you on the road to fulfilling your goals.

What Is the Proper Fitness Walking Form and Technique?

Walking is a natural motion—a movement pattern that most people practice throughout the day. However, many people do not have proper walking form, especially when trying to walk fast enough for fitness.

There are several reasons why people do not walk appropriately. The first reason is poor postural habits and ingrained movement patterns. These habits and patterns are the result of our work environment (slouching at our desks, holding the phone between our ear and shoulder), our home environment (improper lifting and carrying techniques), or life-long poor standing posture. Second, muscle strength and flexibility imbalances can cause irregularities in our stance and gait. Third, in an attempt to walk more vigorously to improve fitness, many people adopt techniques such as an exaggerated arm swing or extra-long strides (called overstriding) that actually slow them down, lead to fatigue, and eventually contribute to athletic injuries.

The following do's and don'ts can help to improve your fitness walking form, comfort level, and performance.

What Leads to Improper Fitness Walking Form?

There are several walking form errors commonly seen in fitness walkers. Read through the following list (paraphrased in part from *The Walking Magazine*, September/October 1996) to determine if you have developed any bad habits:

- Let your elbows flap out to the sides (elbows pointing towards your walking partner)
- Swing your arms rigidly and straight at the elbows
- Let your hips have an exaggerated side-to-side sashay
- Droop or round your shoulders forward (slouching forward)
- Excessively arch your lower back
- Reach forward with your feet to get the longest possible stride (overstriding—a more detailed explanation is provided later in this chapter)
- Swing your hands up above chest height and then drive your elbows back so hard that your hand goes past your waistband, beyond your torso

How Can You Optimize Fitness Walking Form?

Now that you have reviewed everything you shouldn't do while fitness walking, it is time to focus on the do's. The following tips and hints (also paraphrased in part from *The Walking Magazine*, September/October 1996) will help you walk with ease and comfort:

- Stand tall and look forward, not down at the ground
- Relax your neck, back, and shoulders
- Bend your elbows no more than a 90 degree angle
- Have your hands trace an arc from your waistband to chest height
- Gently contract your abdominal and lower back muscles to keep your body erect and stabilized
- Take a comfortable stride so your feet touch down practically beneath you
- Consciously push off with your toes at the end of every step
- Focus on quick, comfortable steps

Source: The Walking Magazine, September/October 1996, p. 72–73

note

A special focus should be placed on maintaining proper form throughout the duration of a long walk or run. As you become fatigued, walking and running form begin to deteriorate.

What Is Racewalking?

Walking activities, including racewalking, have become among the most popular forms of recreation and competition in the world. Racewalking refers to a specific style of walking. Participating and learning to racewalk does not mean you have to race. Anyone can racewalk without feeling the pressure of competition.

What Is the History and Background of Racewalking?

Racewalking events have been part of the Olympic Games since 1908. Distances have been set at 20K (12.4 miles) and 50K (31.1 miles) for men. The 1992 Olympics was the first Olympics to include a racewalking event for women, at the 10K (6.2 miles) distance. In 1999, the distance for women was changed to 20K.

One of the main distinguishing factors of racewalking is the pace of walking. Presently elite male racewalkers average 5:30–5:45 min/mile for the 20K, and women average near 7:00 min/mile for the 10K. Racewalking can be differentiated from strolling or fitness walking by the average minutes/mile or miles per hour:

- Strolling = 20 min/mile or 3mph
- Fitness walking = 15 min/mile or 4mph
- Racewalking = 12 min/mile or 5mph

The rules of the sport also differentiate racewalking from fitness walking. Racewalking is defined by two rules:

1. The lead leg must make contact with the ground before the rear foot leaves the ground (that is, continuous contact) so that no visible loss of contact occurs, to differentiate racewalking from running). If a racewalker violates this rule, it is referred to as *lifting*.

2. The walker must straighten her/his advancing leg from the first moment of contact with the ground (that is, straightened leg, no bent knee) until it is in the vertical upright position (distinguishes racewalking from running and fitness walking). A straight leg does not mean a locked knee; locked joints can cause damage to soft tissues or bones. If a racewalker violates this rule, it is referred to as *creeping*.

Figure 6.1 shows an example of the proper technique (legal racewalking) and examples of improper technique (illegal racewalking) that result in disqualification from a certified racewalking competition. Certified judges observe competitive racewalking events, and when, in the opinion of three different judges, a walker violates either of the two rules, an athlete will be disqualified from the race. As mentioned earlier regarding form, the two infractions are loss of contact lifting or bent knee creeping.

FIGURE 6.1

Legal racewalking form includes keeping one foot in contact with the ground at all times and maintaining a straight leg from the moment of contact with the ground until the leg is in a vertical upright position.

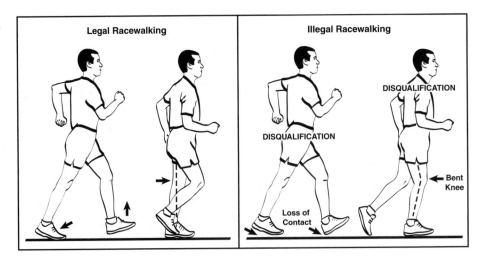

What Is the Proper Racewalking Form and Technique?

Racewalking technique is governed by the rules of the sport and by body mechanics. The following tips provide specific guidelines for developing proper racewalking form:

- *Foot action*—Your driving foot (back foot) and front foot should move in a straight line with full extension and flexion of the ankle joints.

- *Leg action*—Walk with smooth, rhythmic strides ensuring continuous contact with the ground. Maintain a straight lead leg until your leg is in a vertical position beneath your body. Focus on a strong rear leg drive, moving your leg quickly in front of your body in preparation for the next foot strike.

- *Hip action*—Rotate your hips in a smooth forward movement with as little vertical and lateral movement as is necessary.

- *Arm action*—Your hands should come toward the mid-line of your trunk when pumping your arms forward, but not crossing the midline of your body. On the back swing, your arms should move straight back with your elbow high behind your torso. Your arms should be angled at 90 degrees at the elbow.

- *Trunk position*—Your torso should be upright and relaxed, except for a slight lean (5 degrees from the ankle), as your rear leg drives your body forward.

- *Shoulder action*—Keep your shoulders as low as possible and relaxed. Limit side-to-side swaying motions.

- *Head position*—Your head should be upright with your eyes focusing 10–15 feet in front of you, limiting oscillating motions and maintaining relaxed neck muscles.

Figure 6.2 shows the results of putting all the action/position guidelines into practice. The numbers in Figure 6.2 correspond to the descriptions that follow.

FIGURE 6.2
Put the action/position guidelines into practice.

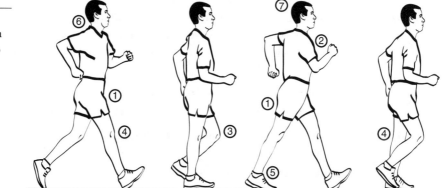

1. Hips drop and roll while twisting back and forth. This allows your legs to move faster and easier, and gives you a longer stride. Note how the stripe on the side of the shorts moves from front to rear, indicating a twisting motion.

2. Arms should always be bent at a 90 degree angle and pumped vigorously. Let them swing across your chest toward, but not past, your trunk midline as they move back and forth.

3. The knee bends as your leg is swung forward. This allows the toes to clear the ground.

4. The knee is straightened from the point of contact with the ground until in a vertical position underneath your body. Your foot should feel like it is "pulling" the ground as your heal touches.

5. Toes and calf muscles push your body forward in a strong driving motion. Feet land in a straight line with the body, and toes are pointed directly forward.

6. Keep your neck and shoulders relaxed.

7. Your trunk and head should be in an upright position at all times.

Concentrate on correct racewalking technique during training and competition. Proper form feels better, prevents injuries, and is required by the rules of the sport during competition to avoid disqualification. Developing proper form will take time, but with regular practice racewalking will begin to feel natural.

How Can Racewalking Drills Improve Your Form?

Racewalking drills are strengthening, stretching, or technique exercises specifically geared toward improving your form. Drills are practiced during your warm-up before completing the workout for the day. Eventually, the techniques emphasized in each drill will transfer into correct body positioning and a smoother stride. The following drills can be practiced several times a week as part of your warm-up. The drills should be done after 5–10 minutes of easy walking and stretching. Begin with two sets of each drill you choose, traveling no further than 10 yards. As you improve and your body adjusts, gradually increase the length from 10 to 40 yards for each drill:

1. *Heel Walk*—Walk on your heels, with your toes pointed up.

    Objective: Strengthens the anterior, or front, part of your lower leg.

2. *Cross Overs*—Walk on a straight line, exaggerating the cross over with your feet, and drop your hand below your knee on the side of the leading leg.

    Objective: Develops hip drop and mobility.

3. *High Knees*—Lift one knee towards your chest while pushing off from the balls of your feet; repeat on each side in a forward walking motion.

   Objective: Develops push off.

4. *Calf Raises*—Stand, using a chair for balance. Raise up on the ball of one foot through a full range of motion, returning to the original position. Repeat with your other leg.

   Objective: Increases calf strength for a strong push off.

5. *Pool Walker*—Keeping your arms down at your side, exaggerate your shoulder and trunk rotation and stride length, while walking forward.

   Objective: Improves hip rotation.

6. *Trunk Stability*—Walk while holding your arms crossed in front of your chest or crossed behind your back. Holding a stick behind your back at waist height or shoulder height can also be used to stabilize your arms while performing this drill.

   Objective: Decreases erratic upper body movements, limits horizontal forces and keeps the upper torso more rigid.

7. *Windmills*—Perform arm circles, keeping your arms straight, slightly brushing your ears when circling. Perform exercises in both forward and backward directions.

   Objective: Develops coordination and decreases shoulder tightness.

8. *Lunges*—Step forward with one leg, allowing the knee of your trailing leg to dip down toward the ground. Repeat with your other leg.

   Objective: Develops quadriceps and hamstring strength.

9. *Quick Steps*—Hold your arms behind your back and racewalk with short, quick steps.

   Objective: Increases leg turnover or stride rate.

note

Practicing proper fitness walking, racewalking, or running form becomes increasingly important as the distance of your training and competitions increases. As you progress towards training for a 10K or half-marathon, proportionately more time during your training should be dedicated to drill and technique exercises.

before you head out the door

Remind yourself to focus on proper form when fitness walking, racewalking, or running. Consider taking time after a 5–10 minute warm-up to practice walking and running drills before completing the scheduled walk or run for the day.

What Is the Proper Running Form and Technique?

One of the keys to distance running is learning how to run efficiently. The more energy you waste by being inefficient, the less energy you will have at the end of a race. The following guidelines can help you properly position your body to be efficient when running short and long distances. Keep in mind that running form contributes only partially to running efficiency. Fitness level, flexibility, strength, and even genetics all play important roles in running efficiency. Please remember the following are only guidelines. Each runner is unique and form will vary. Running form changes may not be necessary for everyone.

How Can You Optimize Your Stride Length?

Stride length is the distance from toe-off to the next contact of the same foot. Generally, a person with a longer stride length uses less energy covering a specified distance than another runner with a shorter stride length. The decreased energy expenditure or exertion makes it feel "easier" to run. To increase stride length, do the following:

- *Increase leg strength and power through strength training.* When your legs are strong and powerful, you can "explode" forward, increasing your stride length.
- *Enhance flexibility by performing stretching exercises on a regular basis.* By increasing the flexibility in your hips, gluteals, hamstrings, and lower back, your stride can naturally lengthen because you have a greater range of motion.
- *Engage in hill training.* Running hills can help to develop more explosive foot-strikes and a longer stride length. Once every one to two weeks, find a hilly course to run, accelerating uphill and then jogging downhill.

While "easy" running sounds good, not everyone should strive for a longer stride. An excessive stride length (overstriding) can be more detrimental to running form than a short stride length. The next section will cover how to prevent overstriding.

How Can You Prevent Overstriding?

Overstriding is defined as the excessive reaching out in front of the body with the feet. It is one of the most common problems in running form. As mentioned in the last section, increasing stride length can lead to faster running times. However, the lengthening should be a result of increasing strength, power, and flexibility in the core and lower body versus trying to force yourself to reach further out in front while running. Ironically, this "forced" reaching out can actually slow runners down by having a braking effect. To reduce overstriding:

- *Do not force yourself to increase stride length.* Avoid reaching out by planting your feet as close to the front of your body as possible, even slightly under the hip.

- *Avoid straightening the knees.* When runners are trying to force a greater stride length, the front legs tends to straighten in attempts to reach further out in front. Your knees should remain slightly bent as they swing through and your feet strike the ground.

- *Engage lower body muscles.* Use your hamstring and gluteal muscles to pull and extend the legs back just prior to the foot strike.

- *Avoid an excessive heel strike.* Runners who hit the pavement hard with their heels also tend to overstride. Aim for a forefoot strike.

How Can You Maintain a High Stride Rate?

Stride rate is the number of foot strikes of one foot in one minute. Stride rate is paramount in determining running efficiency and performance. Research has shown that most top-level runners maintain at least 90 to 95 strides per minute when running 7 minutes/mile or faster. Establish a quick leg turnover and stride rate by

- *Measuring your current stride rate and adapt accordingly.* Count the number of foot strikes of one foot for one minute to establish your baseline stride rate. If your rate is slower than 90–95 strides per minute, aim to increase your leg turnover by moving your legs more rapidly.

- *Engage the hip flexor muscles.* Use the hip flexor muscles (front of the hip) to pull the legs through quickly, increasing leg turnover.

- *Engage hamstring and gluteal muscles.* Use your hamstrings and gluteal muscles to extend the leg forcefully and quickly backward, immediately following the foot strike.

- *Avoid an excessive knee lift.* Lift the knees only high enough for the foot to clear the ground.

Maintaining a high stride rate requires concentration. Leg turnover will slow down as your run progresses if you are not paying attention.

What Is the Proper Running Posture and Arm Swing?

Running posture and arm swing can affect stride length and stride rate. As a runner becomes fatigued, both posture and arm swing can change, affecting overall run form. When running form changes and weakens during a run, undue stress and strain can be placed on the body, potentially leading to injuries. For improved performance and injury prevention, try the following tips to keep your body relaxed and moving forward quickly:

- Posture should be upright or slightly leaned forward just ahead of your center of gravity
- Head should remain stationary and above your center of gravity
- Eyes should be focused 5–10 meters ahead
- Allow your arms to swing naturally in a forward motion, not side to side
- Keep your hips and shoulders square–no twisting
- Shoulders should be loose; face and jaw relaxed
- Arms should bend at 90 degrees
- Elbows move along side your body, thumbs up, hands cupped and relaxed
- Hands should not cross the midline of your body

Strengthening exercises for the upper body, shoulders, and core can help maintain proper posture and arm swing, especially when you are getting fatigued. Refer to Chapter 8, "Strength Training," for strengthening exercises for runners.

What Is Vertical Oscillation?

Vertical oscillation refers to bouncing when running. Studies have shown that highly efficient runners have the least amount of vertical oscillation. Bouncing not only increases the amount of energy expended with each stride, it also increases the impact forces that can lead to injury. To reduce your vertical oscillation or bounce:

- Apply the tips mentioned previously for improving your stride length, stride rate, posture, and arm swing
- Use your hamstrings and gluteal muscles to create horizontal propulsion instead of vertical oscillation

How Should Runners Breathe?

The way you breathe can have a major impact on your running efficiency. As exertion levels rise, the tendency is to tighten the upper body and chest. This results in shallow, tight-chested breathing. This limits the amount of oxygen that can fully perfuse into your lungs, thus limiting performance. In order to maximize your breathing, do the following:

- Relax your upper body
- Use your diaphragm muscle to expand the lungs as you inhale and "squeeze" out unwanted carbon dioxide as you exhale
- You should be able to feel your abdomen protruding as you inhale
- Breathing rate should increase as the intensity level rises

note

To maintain peak efficiency during training and racing, frequently check your form from head to toe. One of the best ways to accurately determine your running form strengths and weaknesses is through a running form/gait analysis conducted by an exercise physiologist or training expert. This test will provide visual feedback of your current running form to help you improve your technique.

How Can Running Drills Improve Your Form?

Running drills are strengthening or technique exercises specifically geared toward improving your form. Drills are practiced during your warm-up, before completing the workout for the day. Eventually, the techniques emphasized in each drill will transfer into correct body positioning and a smoother stride. The following drills can be practiced several times a week as part of your warm up. The drills should be done after 5–10 minutes of easy running and stretching. Begin with two sets of each drill you choose, traveling no further than 10 yards. As you improve and your body adjusts, gradually increase the length from 10 to 40 yards for each drill:

1. *Marching No Arms*—Concentrate on relaxing your upper body, alternate lifting your knees as high as possible, and staying on the balls of your feet. Don't lean back. Avoid twisting at the hips or shoulders. *Remember, knee up, heel up, toe up.*

   Objective: Improved posture, prevents overstriding

2. *Marching with Arms*—Bend your arms at a 90-degree angle at the elbow. As your arm comes forward, the angle of your arm may decrease slightly. Your hand should come to shoulder or mouth level. As your arm moves back, your hand passes the hip. As your arm continues back, the angle of your arm may increase slightly. Your hand should stop approximately one foot behind your body. March with your legs as done in the Marching No Arms drill. *Remember, opposite arm with opposite leg.*

   Objective: Improved posture and arm swing, prevents overstriding

3. *Marching with Bounce ("A" skip)*—Same as "marching with arms" but a short, quick skip is performed with each step forward. Basically, step forward with one foot and hop on that foot once before stepping forward with the other foot. This is a drill involving rhythm.

Objective: Develops strength and power for a strong stride/push-off

4. *Foreleg Reach ("B" Skip)*—Upper body remains relaxed. Lift one knee as performed for "marching." When your knee has reached its highest point, extend your foreleg forward. With the foreleg extended, paw your foot back to the ground directly under your body and repeat with the opposite leg while moving slowly forward. Don't lean back. *Remember, knee up, foreleg reach, paw foot down.*

Objective: Increases stride length

5. *Butt Kicks*—Upper body remains relaxed. Rise onto the balls of your feet. Heels are alternately raised to the buttocks while running *slowly* forward without lifting the knees. Concentrate on keeping your knees pointed down. Don't lift your knees.

Objective: Increases stride rate by teaching "fast feet"

6. *High Knees No Arms*—Upper body remains relaxed. Raise onto the balls of your feet and begin lifting your knees as high and as rapidly as possible while moving slowly forward. This differs from Marching No Arms because you should be moving the legs rapidly. Imagine how a football player runs through tires. *Remember to stay out over the feet. Don't lean back!*

Objective: Increases stride rate

7. *High Knees with Arms*—Legs perform the same movement as in High Knees No Arms, but your arms pump alternately with your legs. Opposite arm with opposite leg. Concentrate on taking small steps forward quickly.

Objective: Promotes correct arm swing and increases stride rate

8. *High Knees Fast Frequency*—Same as the High Knees with Arms drill except that you pump your arms as fast as possible. *Remember, the faster the arms are pumped, the faster the legs move!*

Objective: Promotes correct arm swing and increases stride rate

9. *Back Pedal*—Keep your head up and back straight. Arms swing from the shoulder through a full range of motion, with no twisting of the upper body. Lean forward slightly at the waist, but run tall. Maintain a good cycle action at the hip, knee, and ankle. The knee lift is approximately 45 degrees just before the reach back. Extend fully at the hip to allow for an exaggerated stride length. When the foot of the extended leg makes contact with the

ground, ride the momentum and give a forceful push as your upper body passes over the ground leg.

Objective: Increases stride length

10. *Power Shuffle*—Keep your head up, back straight, knees flexed, and arms slightly bent just below shoulder height. Don't lean forward at the waist. Flex your knees to ensure a low center of gravity. If moving to the right, turn your right foot slightly toward the direction of travel and keep your left foot perpendicular to the direction of travel. Simultaneously push off your left leg while forcefully driving your right knee in the direction of travel. When your right foot makes contact with the ground, pull with your right leg and slide your left foot to the right (don't cross the left foot in front of the right).

Objective: Decreases vertical oscillation

11. *Walking Lunges (Forward and Backward)*—Take one exaggerated step directly forward with the lead leg. Keep your lead knee and foot aligned, and toes pointing straight ahead. Plant the lead foot squarely on floor. Flex the lead knee slowly and with control. Lower the trailing knee toward the floor, but do not let the knee touch the floor. Keep your torso vertical to the floor by "sitting back" on the trailing leg. Keep the lead knee directly over the lead foot. Keep the lead foot flat on floor. Do not bounce in bottom position. Forcefully push off with the lead leg. Bring your trailing foot back to a position next to the lead foot. Alternate lead legs and repeat. *Reverse these directions for backward lunges.*

Objective: Improves lower body strength and control

RUNNING AND WALKING TRAINING GADGETS—RUN/WALK FORM ANALYSIS

For those of you who are serious about improving your running and walking form, I strongly suggest seeking a professional who can observe and critique your form. Often referred to as a *form* or *gait analysis*, you can expect to be videotaped while running or walking on a track or treadmill. Slow motion video analysis allows the professional performing the test to critique your posture, stride length, foot strike, vertical oscillation, pronation, supination, trunk rotation, and arm swing. After identifying your strengths and weaknesses, you can focus your attention on the drills that will be most beneficial to your specific needs. Not only can a running/walking analysis improve your speed and efficiency, but it can also provide insight to the best shoes for your body and form. Check local hospitals, sports medicine facilities and training centers, running/walking shoe stores, and health clubs for exercise science professionals who are experienced in performing form and gait analyses.

In summary, there are many aspects to fitness walking, racewalking, and running form that you can improve to enhance efficiency and make walking and running feel easier. Keep in mind that any modifications involving your form should only be practiced a few minutes a day. Progress slowly and give your body plenty of time to adapt to new movement patterns. It may take months or even a year or two for these changes to feel natural.

THE ABSOLUTE MINIMUM

- Become aware of the strengths and weaknesses of your current walking or running form.
- Practice walking and running form drills to correct your weaknesses.
- Integrate proper technique into your walking and running sessions, being particularly attentive to form as your walks and runs increase in duration.
- Seek the advice of a professional trained in walking and running form/gait analysis. If you have been injured in the past, this can prevent future problems.

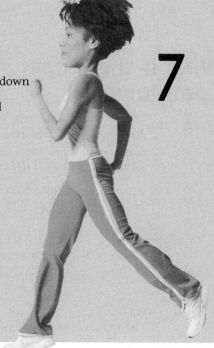

IN THIS CHAPTER

- Guidelines for warming up and cooling down

- Importance of flexibility for runners and walkers

- Various methods of stretching

- Full body, static stretching routine

7

WARM-UP/COOL-DOWN AND FLEXIBILITY EXERCISES

Take time to warm-up, cool-down, and stretch—it's worth it.

Walkers and runners are often so eager to hit the road that they bolt out the door like lightning, moving quickly into their target heart rate zone. Then, in attempts to fit 26 hours worth of work into one day, walkers and runners fly back into the house after their walk or run and rush off to accomplish the next item on their to-do list. If this pattern continues over time, aches, pains, and athletic injuries may begin to emerge; or, even worse, cardiovascular complications may arise. It is worth 10–15 minutes of your time to warm-up, cool-down, and stretch in order to stay safe and healthy, and move forward in your training.

What Is the Proper Way to Warm-Up and Cool-Down?

Prior to beginning any running or walking session you should warm-up for 5–10 minutes. The purpose of a warm-up is to prepare your body—especially your cardiorespiratory and musculoskeletal systems—for activity. Your body needs to warm-up before physical activity, just like your car does before driving.

Warming up is important for a variety of reasons, including the following:

- Allowing your body temperature to increase slightly.
- Loosening up your joints and muscles.
- Allowing your heart and lungs to operate efficiently.
- Reducing the risk of injury.
- Preparing you mentally for the workout to come.

The key to a proper warm-up is to begin slowly, and then gradually increase your intensity over 5–10 minutes. The intensity of your warm-up should progress from very light in the beginning to a gradual ramping up of the intensity to reach the low end of your target heart-rate range at completion. The warm-up movements should be a slower version of the activity you plan to do. For example, walk or jog slowly and then gradually pick up the pace to a brisk walk or run. After your workout, make sure that you cool-down and then stretch.

You should always end a run or walk with 5–10 minutes of cool-down to allow your body to recover. This enables your heart rate, blood pressure, and body temperature to gradually return to a pre-exercise condition. *Never stop exercising suddenly*. Instead continue moving at a slower pace until your body stops sweating. Don't overlook this guideline; cooling down is critical for the prevention of cardiac complications or abnormalities. After your body has sufficiently cooled down, it is time to stretch.

before you head out the door

Make sure to take time to warm-up sufficiently before increasing the intensity of your walk or run. Before you begin, remind yourself to go easy at first, slowly working into the specified workout for the day.

Why Is Flexibility Important to Runners and Walkers?

Flexibility is the range of motion (ROM) possible in a joint or a series of joints.

Maintaining flexibility facilitates movement in all joints within the body, especially while running or walking. Stretching exercises are the main avenues to increasing flexibility. There are many benefits to engaging in a regular stretching program to maintain or improve flexibility, including the following:

■ *Reducing muscle tension and increasing relaxation.* As with any type of exercise, stretching can be an excellent stress management and relaxation tool. Stretching can help alleviate pain and soreness due to inflexible muscles.

■ *Improving coordination.* Flexibility, especially in opposing muscle groups, can facilitate coordination with any bodily movement.

■ *Improvement and development of body awareness.* Body awareness is vital for maintaining proper form while running or walking, as well as establishing spatial orientation with your environment—that is, safely stepping over curbs, logs, cracks in the road, and so forth.

■ *Promoting circulation.* Stretching promotes circulation throughout the body, bringing oxygenated blood to muscles and tissues.

■ *Increasing athletic performance.* Greater flexibility, especially in the hips, knees, and shoulders, can enhance performance in sports that mainly use these joints, such as running and walking.

■ *Preventing injury.* A consistent, regular stretching routine can help prevent injuries on a long-term basis.

■ *Decreasing muscle soreness.* Some research has shown that a cool-down with stretching can decrease post-exercise muscle soreness.

■ *It feels good!*

Flexibility is one of five components that help define overall fitness; the other four include cardiorespiratory endurance, muscular strength and endurance, and body composition (see Figure 7.1). If you are starting a running or walking program with the goal of increasing fitness, you should include flexibility exercises in your weekly exercise routine.

FIGURE 7.1

Components of overall fitness.

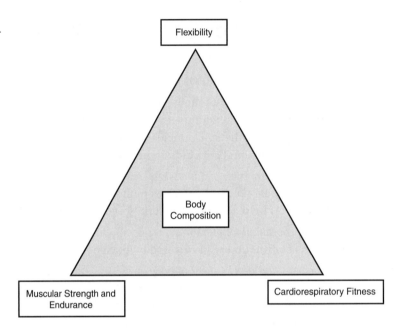

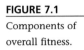

WHO SHOULD NOT STRETCH?

The following people should not stretch:

- Individuals who are hypermobile (excessive range of motion within one joint) should not stretch to extremes.
- Individuals who have unhealed fractures or acute joint inflammation should not stretch the affected areas.
- Individuals who experience sharp pain while stretching should stop the exercise immediately or modify the stretch to avoid pain.

Runners and walkers should engage in some form of stretching on a regular basis. Exercises can be performed in a variety of ways; therefore, you have some flexibility (pun intended) regarding how you stretch. In the next section, you will review a few of the most common ways to increase flexibility through stretching.

What Are Some Common Types of Beneficial Stretching Exercises for Runners and Walkers?

There are many ways to stretch—some are safe and effective, and others are not. Three of the most common ways to stretch, which are safe and effective, include *traditional static stretching, active isolated stretching,* and *yoga.* One or more of these methods should be practiced at least three times a week, but preferably everyday.

A form of stretching that is not safe is *ballistic stretching*. Ballistic stretching involves rapid, repetitive movements, requiring jerking and often bouncing movements. When performing this type of stretch, tissues are rapidly stretched and immediately relaxed. When this happens, the muscle's natural response is to protect itself by quickly contracting to prevent tearing of the muscle tissue. While an important protective reflex, it prevents the muscle from enhancing its flexibility and the joint's range of motion. Additionally, the jerking and tugging of the muscle predisposes tissues to damage. Hence, ballistic stretching is neither safe nor effective and therefore is *not recommended.*

What Is Traditional Static Stretching?

Traditional static stretching involves slowly stretching tissues to enhance your flexibility.

The stretch is held for a period of time, typically 10–30 seconds, and then the tissues are allowed to return to their resting length. Several stretches may be performed on the same muscle group in succession. Static stretching should be slow and gradual— no bouncing is involved. Rather, you move into the stretch until you feel a slight resistance; at that point, hold the stretch for 10–30 seconds, and then relax. Static stretching is appealing to runners and walkers because the stretches can be performed alone, a wide variety of exercises are easy to learn, and it is safe and effective.

The full-body stretching routine presented at the end of this chapter involves only static stretches.

What Is Active Isolated Stretching?

Active isolated stretching involves dynamic, not static, stretches. Dynamic means movement—muscles are stretched and relaxed in a successive and controlled fashion. Do not confuse the terms ballistic and dynamic: Ballistic stretching involves sudden, jerky movements leading to a contractile response by the muscle; dynamic involves smooth contractions and relaxations.

One of the main concepts behind active isolated stretching is that a muscle either contracts *or* relaxes. If ballistic stretching causes a muscle to contract to protect itself, it is impossible for it to also stretch and lengthen. On the other hand, if a muscle can relax through smooth, controlled movements (as suggested through active isolated stretching), it can lengthen, ultimately improving flexibility. The smooth movements during active isolated stretching also promote blood flow through the muscles and surrounding tissues, potentially enhancing the recovery process following running and walking by eliminating waste products.

There are several basic principles to active isolated stretching:

- *Identifying the muscle to be stretched.* Active isolated stretching focuses on specifying the muscle you're stretching; therefore, the first step is to identify the targeted muscle.

- *Isolating the muscle by localized movement.* Using specific form and technique, active isolated stretching focuses on one muscle or muscle group at a time.

- *Intensifying the stretch by contracting the opposite muscle group.* By actively contracting the muscle that is opposite of the targeted muscle, you will cause the targeted muscle to relax and lengthen. For example, when performing a hamstring stretch (back of the thigh), you should actively contract your quadriceps (front of the thigh) to relax your hamstrings and allow for enhanced lengthening.

Because of the specific nature of this type of stretching, it is recommended that you learn more about the concept and appropriate stretches before attempting it on your own. Information can be obtained by visiting active isolated stretching web sites (www.stretchingusa.com; www.aistretch.com), reading an active isolated stretching book, or finding a therapist in your area who is certified to teach and perform active isolated stretching. By scheduling a private session with a certified therapist, you can learn with a hands-on approach, and then perform stretches daily on your own. The www.stretchingusa.com web site can help you find a certified professional in your area.

What Is Yoga?

Yoga was developed in India and has been evolving for about 5,000 years. Yoga actually encompasses an entire lifestyle and belief system; however, most Americans recognize only the physical component of this lifestyle as "yoga." Yoga has many parallels to running and walking including flexibility, strength, and proper breathing. Yoga exercises focus on the entire body, providing a well-balanced workout for walkers and runners who tend to focus only on their lower bodies. Yoga involves performing a combination of stretching and strengthening postures, breathing exercises, and meditation. Yoga can be practiced in a group setting or in the privacy of your home. Check your local gyms for yoga classes for beginners. Also inquire at running/walking or athletic stores—many commercial stores are now offering yoga classes onsite. Many high quality and reputable videos and books are on the market, including versions geared specifically for runners and walkers. Visit www.yoga.com for a sampling of yoga books, videos, and other products.

An added benefit of yoga is the mental focus, meditation, and relaxation practiced during classes. Mental energy is as critical as physical energy for runners and walkers training for all distances. Positive mental energy enables runners and walkers to train consistently, leading to improved performance and the realization of goals.

RUNNING AND WALKING TRAINING GADGETS—STRETCHING TOOLS

If you are interested in trying active isolated stretching or yoga in addition to traditional static stretching, the following products would be helpful. All descriptions taken directly from the products' websites.

Active isolated stretching: Stretching Rope (www.stretchingusa.com)—When performing active isolated stretches on your own, you need a rope to maintain proper form and technique. This 100% nylon rope is durable enough for daily stretching. The rope is eight feet long making stretching easy and comfortable.

Yoga: Tapas Yoga Mat (www.yoga.com)—Practicing yoga on a hard wood floor, tile, or even carpet can be challenging because the slippery nature of the surface. This stable, non-slip mat will provide comfort and security during any yoga class or video.

How Do You Exercise for a Full-Body Stretching Routine?

After you have properly warmed up for 5–10 minutes, or after a workout, it is important to stretch your major muscle groups (the legs, back, chest, shoulders, and arms). Regular stretching can help reduce injuries, relieve muscle soreness and cramps, lessen the possibility of low back pain, and promote relaxation. Almost everyone can feel more flexible by stretching at least three times a week.

To implement an effective static stretching routine, review the following guidelines established by the American College of Sports Medicine:

- Stretch after a 5–10 minute warm-up, or after your workout session once your cool-down is complete.

- Perform stretching exercises for all major muscle groups at least two or three days a week.

- Stretch until the point of mild tension and then hold the stretch for a minimum of 10–30 seconds, or as long as it feels comfortable. Repeat the same stretch three to four times.

- Stretching should be relaxing. Breathe deeply and try to exhale completely as you stretch. Deep breathing will help relax your muscles and calm your mind after a workout.

■ Do not bounce or jerk when stretching.

■ Never force a muscle to stretch past its natural limit. As you stretch, you should feel an awareness of the muscle and mild discomfort, but no pain.

It is important to incorporate both upper and lower body stretches into your routine. Running and walking primarily rely on the torso and lower body for locomotion; however, the upper back, shoulders, and arms play a supporting role in maintaining proper form and therefore deserve equal stretching attention. When performing any stretch, be sure that you are executing the stretch with proper form to prevent any undue strain on muscles or joints.

What Are Four Basic Stretches for the Upper Body?

There are many upper body stretches for improving flexibility in the back, shoulders, arms, and torso. The following sections describe four basic stretches that target the main areas that you use during running and walking. When performing these stretches, keep in mind the following form and technique guidelines:

■ Stand with your knees slightly bent.

■ Your feet should be shoulder-width apart.

■ Your upper body should be aligned with your pelvis.

How Do You Do Arm Circles?

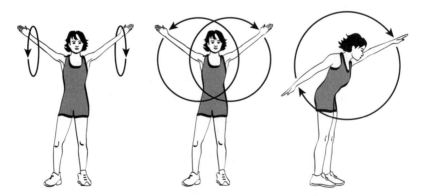

1. Stand with your feet apart, slightly wider than shoulder-width, knees slightly bent and arms at your side.

2. On each of the following arm stretches, swing your arms slowly with large, sweeping circles. Swing your arms from the shoulders and keep your elbows straight, but not locked.

■ *Inward Circles.* Swing your arms inward, crossing in front of your body, moving upward, and over your head; repeat 10–15 times.

■ *Outward Circles.* Swing your arms outward, crossing in front of your body, moving upward, and over your head; repeat 10–15 times.

■ *Forward Circles.* Swing your arms alternately forward, with large sweeping circles, as if swimming. Count one complete circle with the left and right arm as one repetition; repeat 10–15 times.

■ *Backward Circles.* Swing your arms alternately backward, with large sweeping circles. Count one complete circle with the left and right arm as one repetition; repeat 10–15 times.

How Do You Do a Shoulder Stretch?

1. Stand or sit with your right arm across your chest.

2. Grasp your arm just above or below the elbow with your left hand.

3. Gently pull your right arm further across your chest with your left hand.

4. Do not rotate your trunk in the direction of the stretch.

5. Hold for 10–30 seconds.

6. Repeat with your left arm, relax, and repeat two to three times with each arm.

How Do You Do a Triceps Stretch?

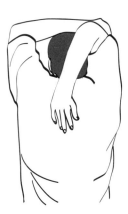

1. While you stand or sit, raise your right arm over your head.

2. Bend at the elbow and place your right hand on your back between your shoulder blades.

3. Grasp your right elbow with your left hand.

4. Gently pull your right elbow behind your head and downward.

5. Hold for 10–30 seconds.

6. Repeat with your left arm, relax, and repeat 2–3 times with each arm.

How Do You Do a Side Stretch?

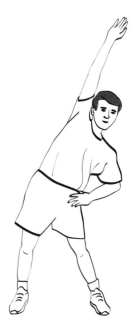

1. Stand with your feet apart, slightly wider than shoulder-width, knees slightly bent, and toes pointing straight ahead.

2. Place your left hand on your left hip for support.

3. Lift your right arm up in line with your right ear and reach upward as high as possible.

4. Continue the stretch by arching your torso further to the left. Be sure to stretch from the side and not twist at the waist.

5. Hold for 10–30 seconds.

6. Return your arms to the side and repeat with your left arm overhead, relax, and repeat two to three times with each arm.

What Are Six Basic Stretches for the Lower Body?

Similar to the upper body stretches, there are many static stretches that can be performed to enhance your lower body flexibility. The following sections describe six basic stretches that target the major lower-body muscle groups used by walkers and runners.

How Do You Do a Hip Twist and Gluteal Stretch?

1. Sit with your legs straight and your upper body nearly vertical; place your right foot on the left side of your left knee.

2. Place the back of your left elbow on the right side of your right knee, which is now bent.

3. Stabilize your upper body with your right hand placed 6–12 inches behind your right hip.

4. Gently push your right knee to the left with your left elbow while turning your shoulders and head to the right as far as possible.

5. Hold for 10–30 seconds.

6. Repeat with your left leg, relax, and repeat two to three times for each side.

How Do You Do a Lower Back and Gluteal Stretch?

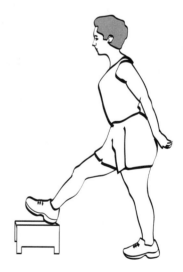

1. Lie on your back with both legs extended while pressing your lower back to the floor.

2. Bend your left knee, grasp behind your knee, and pull it towards your chest, while keeping your head on the floor.

3. Hold for 10–30 seconds, and then curl your shoulders and lift your head and shoulders towards your knee.

4. Hold for 10 seconds.

5. Lower your shoulders and then lower your left leg back to the floor and repeat with your right leg; relax, and repeat two to three times for each leg.

How Do You Do a Hamstring Stretch?

1. Stand with one foot propped up off the ground with your toes pointed up, while the other leg is slightly bent and facing forward.

2. Keep your back straight (flat) and lean forward from the hips.

3. Hold for 10–30 seconds.

4. Alternate legs, relax, and repeat two to three times for each leg.

How Do You Do a Quadriceps Stretch?

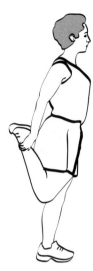

1. Stand on your left leg, holding onto a wall or fixed object with your left hand.

2. Bend your right knee and grasp your right ankle with your right hand, knee pointing down.

3. Slowly pull your right heel towards your buttocks. Do not pull on your ankle so hard that you feel pain or discomfort in the knee.

4. Keep your back straight and stand tall.

5. Hold for 10–30 seconds.

6. Repeat with your left leg; relax, and repeat two to three times for each leg.

note

The quadriceps stretch may be easier to perform while lying on your side.

How Do You Do a Groin Stretch?

1. Sit with your upper body nearly vertical and your legs straight and bend both knees as the soles of your feet come together.

2. Grasp your ankles and pull your feet towards your body.

3. Place your hands on your feet and elbows on your thighs.

4. While keeping your back straight, pull your torso slightly forward as your elbows push your thighs down.

5. Hold for 10–30 seconds, relax, and repeat two to three times.

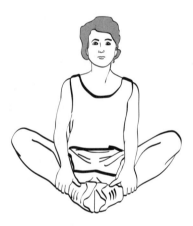

How Do You Do a Gastrocnemius and Soleus Stretch?

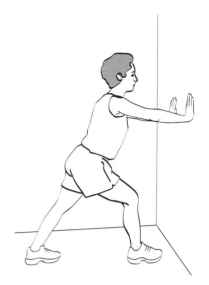

1. Stand facing a wall or other solid support. Place your outstretched hands or forearms on the wall.

2. Place your left leg behind your right leg, keeping your left leg straight.

3. Slowly move your hips and upper torso forward, keeping your back straight, and the heel of your left foot on the ground (this stretches your gastrocnemius).

4. Hold for 10–30 seconds.

5. Now, slowly begin to lower your body a few inches by bending your left knee and keeping the heel of both feet on the ground (this stretches your soleus).

6. Hold for 10–30 seconds.

7. Repeat with the right leg behind the left; relax, and repeat two to three times for each leg.

THE ABSOLUTE MINIMUM

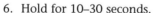

- Warm up for 5–10 minutes by walking or jogging slowly before you increase the intensity to reach your target heart rate range during a workout.

- Cool down for 5–10 minutes after a run or walk to bring your heart rate, blood pressure, and respiration rate back to their baselines.

- Perform stretching exercises on a regular basis—at least two to three times a week, but preferably everyday.

- Try various safe and effective methods of stretching, such as static stretching, active isolated stretching, or yoga, to determine the best fit for you.

- Stretch all major muscle groups in your body.

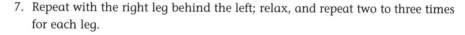

IN THIS CHAPTER

- Benefits of strength training for walkers and runners

- Tailoring a strength training program to fit your needs

- Sample strength training exercises at home and in a gym

- Non-traditional methods of strength training

8

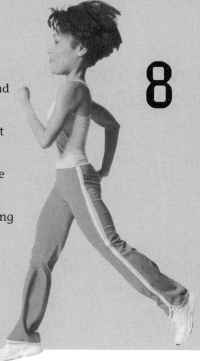

STRENGTH TRAINING

Muscular strength and endurance are essential for healthy walking and running.

Walkers and runners often view pumping iron as important only for body builders and football players. The reality is that *strength training* (also referred to as *resistance training*) is important for everyone—athletes and non-athletes, walkers and runners, body builders and football players. Strength training enhances muscular endurance, allowing you to walk or run further and more comfortably. It also keeps your muscles, joints, and ligaments strong, decreasing your risk for injury while walking and running. In addition to the athletic benefits, strength training keeps your body healthy, functional, and disease-free. So walk or run to your closest gym and start pumping some iron!

How Is Strength Training Beneficial for Runners and Walkers?

Often walkers and runners develop tunnel vision, centering their entire fitness program on cardiorespiratory exercise. Although cardiorespiratory exercise, such as walking and running, is extremely beneficial to the heart, lungs, and body, strength training and stretching are equally as important. Runners and walkers can reap the following benefits by engaging in a regular strength training program:

- *Avoid muscle loss*—Adults who do not strength train lose five to seven pounds of muscle every 10 years. Although walking and running are good cardiorespiratory exercises, they do not promote an increase in muscle tissue and strength, therefore accelerating muscle atrophy with age.

- *Keep metabolism elevated*—Muscle is extremely metabolically active. A person who has more muscle tissue (lean body mass) will have a higher metabolism, even at rest, than a sedentary individual. Metabolism is the rate at which the body burns calories. Without regular strength training, metabolism declines about 2%–5% each year. Strength training prevents muscle loss, which keeps metabolism elevated.

- *Increase strength and functional ability*—Weight training will increase the strength of not only muscles, but tendons and ligaments as well. It has been found that individuals who weight train have more muscle-skeletal control than those who only perform aerobic activity or are sedentary. An increase in muscle control creates more stability especially during weight-bearing activities such as walking and running.

- *Increase bone density*—Resistance training has been shown to increase bone mineral density within a few months of initiating a program. Weight training is especially important for women of all ages to reduce their risk of osteoporosis.

- *Reduce body fat*—As mentioned previously, the more muscle you have, the higher your metabolism and the more calories you burn, ultimately lowering body fat stores. For example, an increase of only 7.7% in the resting metabolic rate of a 180-pound person can result in an increase of 50,000 calories expended yearly. This can result in a 14-pound loss of fat, even if diet and daily physical activity remain constant!

- *Improve athletic performance*—Strength training can enhance your walking and running performance in two ways: by strengthening your muscles, tendons, and ligaments, your risk for athletic-related injuries will decrease; by improving muscle endurance, you will be able to keep walking and running for longer periods of time. These factors are important when training for any distance race, but they become increasingly critical for those of you training for a half-marathon.

Other benefits of strength training include enhanced quality of sleep, reduced depression, and improved digestion. Strength training should be considered equally as important as walking and running and should be incorporated into your weekly training regimen.

What Do You Need to Consider Before Starting a Strength Training Program?

Now that you are excited about reaping the benefits of strength training, take a minute to answer the questions in the following sections.

What Are Your Objectives?

To tailor a program that fits your needs, you should first determine what you want to achieve through engaging in strength training. Do you want to:

- Change your body composition by increasing muscle mass and decreasing fat mass?
- Increase your muscle tone or shape your body?
- Increase your muscle strength?
- Correct a muscle weakness or imbalance?
- Prevent reoccurring injuries?
- Enhance your walking or running performance?

Determine your objectives before reading the rest of this chapter. Your objectives and expected outcomes will influence the development or your program.

My objectives and expected outcomes from engaging in a regular strength-training program include:

- _____
- _____
- _____

Do You Have Any Medical or Orthopedic Concerns That May Be Worsened Through Strength Training?

As with any exercise program, you need to consider how your current or past medical history may affect your ability to perform strength training exercises. Check with your physician before starting a strength training program, especially if you have:

- Uncontrolled high blood pressure
- Uncontrolled diabetes
- Acute musculoskeletal problems or injuries
- History of heart attack or stroke

Also consider the effects of your daily medications; talk to your doctor about how your current medications might affect your ability to strength train.

How Much Time Do You Have Available Each Week to Strength Train?

Training for a 5K, 10K, or half-marathon should be your hobby—not your full-time job. You need to budget your time accordingly for both walking/running and strength training. In order to gain the benefits from strength training, you need to commit to at least two sessions of 30–40 minutes each week. You can complete a full-body routine in 30–40 minutes, targeting all the major muscle groups. If you have less time in a day, but can strength train more frequently, a split routine might be better option. In this scenario, you would engage in strength training exercises four to five times per week, only working a couple of muscle groups in each session, targeting the entire body over the course of a week.

Circle the option that best suits your needs:

I have _____ days per week to dedicate to strength training:

- 2–3
- 4–5

I have _____ minutes in one exercise session to devote to strength training:

- 30–40 minutes for an entire body workout
- 10–20 minutes for multiple split routines

Now that you have determined your main objectives for strength training, talked to your doctor about safety precautions based on your medical history and medications, and committed to at least two days a week, you are ready to begin planning your program.

What Are the Commonly Used Strength Training Terms?

In order to fully comprehend how to develop a strength training program, you need to review the definition of several commonly used terms.

What Is a Repetition?

A *repetition* is one movement through an exercise-specific range of motion. For each exercise, you will perform a series of repetitions in a row. The number of repetitions completed will be determined by your goals and objectives for strength training. Refresh your memory on the objectives you documented earlier in this chapter before reading the rest of this chapter. In general, if your goals are endurance, you should aim for 10–20 repetitions per exercise; if your goals are for strength and building muscle mass, you should aim for 6–10 repetitions per exercise.

What Is a Set?

A *set* is a series of repetitions performed in a sequence. For each exercise, you will perform several sets. The number of sets and the rest in between sets will be determined by your goals and objectives. For example, if your goals are for increased muscular endurance, your rest period in between sets will be 30–60 seconds. If your goals are for strength and muscle building, your rest periods may last several minutes.

What Is a Concentric Contraction?

A *concentric contraction* is the shortening of the muscle during a repetition. You may also hear training partners refer to concentric contractions as the "positive" portion of the movement. For example, when doing a bicep curl, the concentric contraction is when you are bending at the elbow and raising the dumbbell toward your shoulder.

What Is an Eccentric Contraction?

An *eccentric contraction* is the lengthening of the muscle during a repetition. Considered the opposite of a concentric contraction, eccentric contractions are often termed the "negative" portion of the movement. The eccentric contraction of a bicep curl is when you are lowering the weight from shoulder height and straightening your arms.

What Is Muscle Strength?

Muscle strength is the ability of the muscles to contract maximally one time, or the maximum amount you can lift. The prescription for increasing strength is to use heavier weights and lower repetitions; for example, lifting a specific weight a maximum of four to six times.

There are many benefits of developing strong muscles. Muscle strength is important when walking and running up hills and in strong head winds. Muscle strength will help to improve your posture, which will increase your walking and running efficiency. Strength is also vital for supporting your body and preventing injuries in daily living as well as while walking and running. However, performing a routine geared solely for improving strength year-round can be intense and may cause muscle soreness and decreased speed in an upcoming race. Therefore, the best time to work on gaining strength is in your "off-season" when you are not simultaneously engaging in frequent or long-distance walking and running sessions.

What Is Muscle Endurance?

Muscle endurance is the ability of the muscles to repeatedly contract. Essentially, this is how many times you can lift a particular weight. Muscular endurance is best built by lifting a moderate weight using higher repetitions, usually 10–20. To build a combination of strength and endurance, work in the 8–12 repetition range.

Muscle endurance is the basis of walking and running. In order to keep moving, you need to have muscle endurance. This becomes increasingly important as you progress from training for a 5K to a half-marathon. You will be contracting the same muscles repeatedly for at least 20 to 30 minutes (for those training for a 5K) to upwards of three to four hours (for those of you training for a half-marathon). Performing exercises to improve your muscular endurance will greatly enhance your walking and running abilities. Muscle endurance can be targeted year-round, especially during "in-season" time when you are training for your 5K, 10K, or half-marathon.

What Is Progressive Overload?

Progressive overload refers to the fact that strength, endurance, and size of a muscle will increase only when stimulated at workloads above those normally experienced by the muscle tissue. In other words, you need to change your routine every four to eight weeks to continue to challenge your muscles to improve. Your body will adapt to the stress of a strength training program over the course of several weeks. You will know when your body has adapted because the exercises will become "easy" to complete. When you realize that the exercises are no longer challenging, you need to either aim for more repetitions within a set of a specific exercise, or increase the weight and attempt to complete the same number of repetitions. Without progressively overloading your muscles, you will not improve and you will be wasting your time in the gym. You do not need to wait until the four to eight week mark before changing the number of repetitions or sets for a specific exercise—do that whenever an exercise becomes "easy." When you do reach four to eight weeks, change your program to incorporate 8 to 10 new exercises, as well as potentially a different number of sets and repetitions.

What Are the Eight "Rules to Lift By?"

There are several basic rules to follow when performing any strength training exercise. These rules have been developed to ensure that you have a safe and effective workout:

1. **One repetition maximal lifts should be avoided**. It increases your risk of injury and provides little benefit to the walker or runner.

2. **Warm-up** for weight training by doing 5–10 minutes of light cardiorespiratory exercise or do a couple of light warm-up sets of the exercise you plan to do. The warm-up increases blood flow, deep muscle temperature, and neurological recruitment of the muscle fibers.

3. After weight training during the cool-down, **stretch** to quicken recovery, increase flexibility, and aid in injury prevention.

4. It is important to **breathe** properly when strength training. In weight training, you should exhale on the exertion phase of the movement. Be sure to breathe with every repetition. *Do not hold your breath while performing exercises.*

5. Work through a **full range of motion** without hyperextending any joint. Lifting a weight through a full range of motion develops strength at various angles of movement allowing for the application of exercises in the gym to transfer to real-life situations. For example, when performing a squat, your back should be straight while you "sit back" until the point at which your knees are near a 90 degree angle, and then return to a standing position. This movement is exactly what should happen when you lift a box: back is straight, bend at the knees (instead of bending from the waist) and use your legs to lift the box (instead of lifting with your back). If you were to perform your squat with a limited range of motion, you would not have trained your muscles to be strong and controlled from the time you squat down to pick up the box to the point of full extension, box in-hand.

6. Use **smooth, controlled movements**. Avoid lifting too fast, where the momentum controls the movement.

7. Exercise all body parts. Your program must be **balanced** to prevent injuries. A balanced program incorporates 8–10 different exercises targeting the major muscles groups of the body. Without a balanced program, strength training will lead to the over-development of a muscle group, which can lead to injury.

8. Avoid being over-competitive with others. **Do not measure your strength gains or physique against others.** Genetics plays an important part of our strength potential.

How Can You Tailor a Strength Training Program to Fit Your Needs?

Now that you have established your objectives and checked with your physician regarding medical clearance to begin a strength training program, it is time to put a program together that will meet your needs. The American College of Sports Medicine (ACSM) has issued some basic guidelines to follow when developing a plan. These recommendations are based on the frequency, intensity, duration, and mode of strength training that research has shown will elicit the benefits stated earlier in this chapter. The ACSM guidelines are shown in Figure 8.1.

FIGURE 8.1

Use these guidelines when developing your strength training program.

American College of Sports Medicine	
Resistance Training Program Guidelines	
Source: ACSM's Guidelines for Exercise Testing and Prescription, 6th Edition, 2000	
Frequency	perform exercises 2-3 times per week
Intensity	moderate, but challenging; each set should be performed until the point of volitional fatigue*
Duration	perform at least 1 set of 8-12 repetitions for each exercise. For those primarily interested in improving endurance, 10-15 repetitions might be more appropriate
Mode	perform a minimum of 8-10 separate exercises focuses on the major muscle groups including arms, shoulders, chest, back, abdomen, hips and legs; a single session should last no longer than 45-60 minutes

* volitional fatigue means that the final repetition of the set is the last one you can do while maintaining proper form. The final repetition of each set and every exercise should feel very challenging to complete. This ensures you are taxing your muscles enough to stimulate improvement in your muscle endurance, strength, and size. If it feels easy at the end of the set, increase the number of repetitions or increase the weight.

Building on the ACSM recommendations, the chart shown in Figure 8.2 provides information on how to specifically design a program, factoring in all the variables mentioned previously in this chapter. Realizing that some of you may currently be engaging in a regular strength training program, the chart provides information that allows everyone to begin at an appropriate stage as well as progress over the course of 13 weeks. For first timers, follow the initial conditioning schedule; if you have been strength training for one or two months, begin with the intermediate conditioning recommendations; and if strength training is old hat to you, being at the advanced conditioning stage. Upcoming sections within this chapter will provide examples of exercises for all the major muscle groups that can be performed at a gym or in your home.

FIGURE 8.2

Designing your strength training program.

Stage	Choice of Exercises	Order of Exercises	Number of Sets	Number of Repetitions	Load (intensity)	Rest Periods
Initial Conditioning (first 4-6 weeks)	1 exercise per body part: compound movements†	**For all stages:** 1. large before small muscle groups	1-2 sets per exercise	10-12 for upper body exercises; 15-20 for lower body exercises	**For all stages:** weight should be adjusted to allow	60 seconds between sets
Intermediate Conditioning (7-12 weeks)	2 exercises per body part: compound movements	2. Compound before simple movements	2-3 sets per exercise	6-8 strength and 10-12 endurance for upper body; 8-10 strength and 15-20 endurance for lower body	for the desired number of repetitions to be completed to	60-90 seconds for endurance; 90-120+ seconds for strength
Advanced Conditioning (13+ weeks)	2-3 exercises per body part: 2 compound movements, 1 simple movement*	3. Lower back and abdominal exercises should be performed last	2-4 sets per exercise	Same as intermediate	volitional fatigue for each set.	Same as intermediate

† compound movements: exercises involving multiple muscle groups (i.e., leg press)

* simple movements: exercises involving only one muscle group (i.e., bicep curl)

What Are Some Basic Strength Training Exercises You Can Perform at the Gym?

Each fitness center has a different line of strength training equipment. The following exercises are based on Cybex-Eagle equipment. If your gym has a different set of machines, ask a fitness instructor at your facility to help you locate the machines that would work the same muscle groups as listed in the following sections.

Before using the Cybex-Eagle, or any other type of strength training equipment, adjust the various settings of each machine for a proper individual fit. If you are unsure of how to make the correct adjustments, ask a fitness instructor on-site who can provide guidance. Remember to lift the weights in a controlled and steady manner, lifting on a two count and lowering on a four count. Also, remember to exhale when exerting (lifting) and inhale when lowering the weight.

Multi-Hip

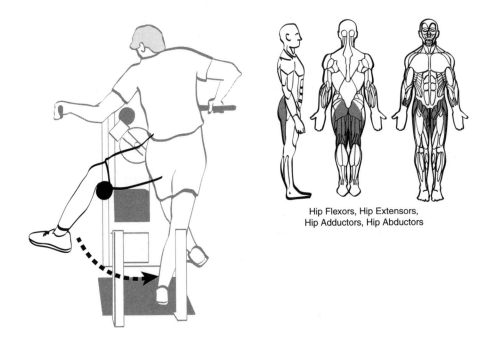

Hip Flexors, Hip Extensors,
Hip Adductors, Hip Abductors

Objective: To strengthen the hip flexors, hip extensors, hip adductors, and hip abductors.

1. Adjust the height of the platform (your hip joint should be aligned with the axis of the pivot arm).

2. Adjust the position of the leg pad (position the pad just above your knee joint).

3. Select the exercise (hip flexion, extension, adduction, or abduction).

4. Position the joint involved to align with the axis of the pivot arm and grasp the handles for stabilization.

5. Lift and lower the weight with smooth, controlled movements.

Leg Extension

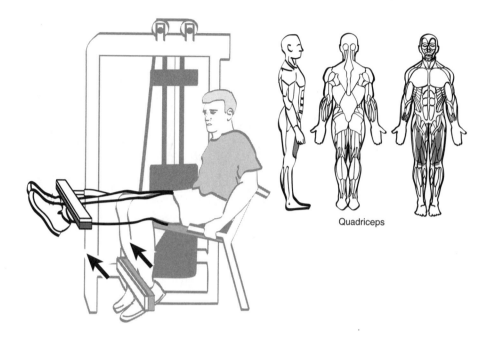

Quadriceps

Objective: To strengthen the quadriceps.

1. Adjust the leg pad (position the pad above your ankles).
2. Adjust the back pad (your knee joint should be aligned with the axis of the cam).
3. Grip the handles lightly.
4. Lift and lower the weight with smooth, controlled movements.

Chest Press

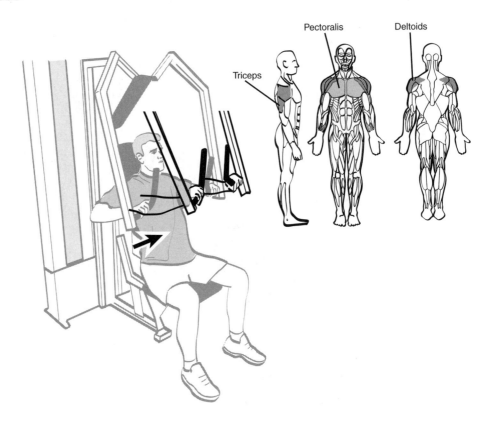

Objective: To strengthen the triceps, deltoids, and pectoralis.

1. Adjust the seat height (the handles should be even with your sternum).
2. Select a grip (neutral or barbell).
3. Lift-lower the weight with smooth, controlled movements.

Pullover

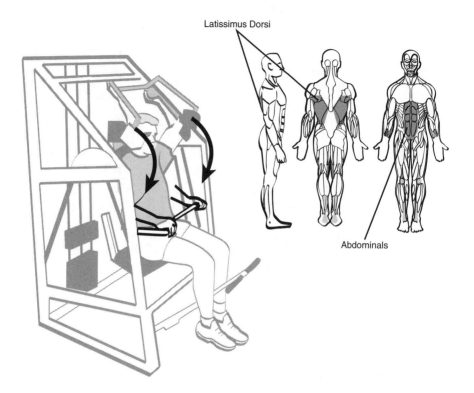

Latissimus Dorsi

Abdominals

Objective: To strengthen the latissimus dorsi and the abdominals.

1. Adjust the seat height (your shoulder joint should be aligned with the axis of the cam).
2. Use the foot pedal to advance the arm handles.
3. Keep a light grip on the exercise bar (push with your elbows).
4. Lift and lower the weight with smooth, controlled movements.
5. Use the foot pedals to return the weight to the starting position and exit the machine.

Rowing

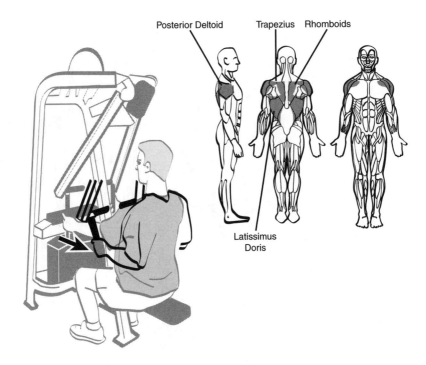

Objective: To strengthen the posterior deltoid, trapezius, rhomboids, and latissimus dorsi.

1. Adjust the seat height (your arms should be parallel with the floor).
2. Adjust the chest pad (to allow your arms to fully straighten during the exercise).
3. Select a grip (neutral or barbell).
4. Lift and lower the weight with smooth, controlled movements.

Shoulder Press

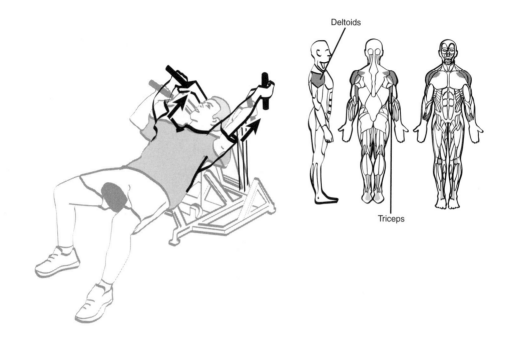

Objective: To strengthen the deltoids and triceps.

1. Adjust the seat height (the handles should be level with the top of your shoulders).
2. Select a grip (neutral or barbell).
3. Lift-lower the weight with smooth, controlled movements.

Triceps Press

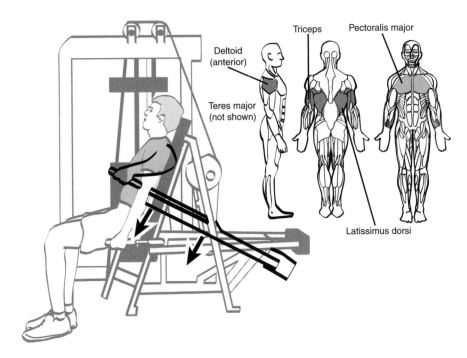

Objective: To strengthen the anterior deltoids, pectoralis major, teres major, triceps, and latissimus dorsi.

1. Adjust the seat height (corresponding to the desired range of motion).

2. Adjust the grips to a wide or narrow position.

3. Fasten the seat belt.

4. Lift and lower the weight with smooth, controlled movements.

Abdominal

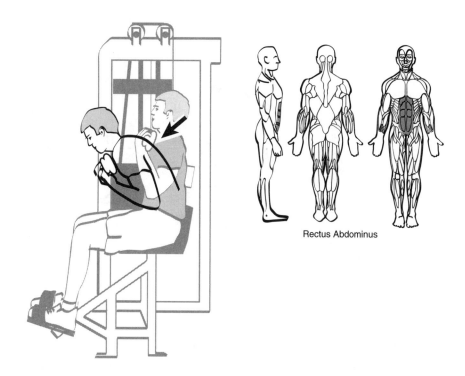

Rectus Abdominus

Objective: To strengthen the rectus abdominus.

1. Adjust the seat height (align the chest pad just below your clavicle).
2. Adjust the height of the front foot plate (your upper and lower leg should form a 90 degree angle).
3. Secure your feet under the instep straps or behind the instep pads.
4. Place your hands on top of your thighs or on the exercise bar.
5. Lift and lower the weight with smooth, controlled movements.

Back Extension

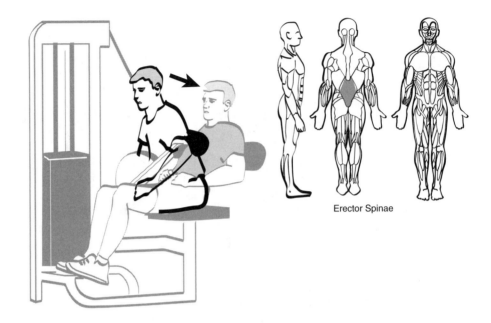

Erector Spinae

Objective: To strengthen the erector spinae.

1. Adjust the foot plate (your hips should be aligned with the axis of the machine, with your knees bent slightly).

2. Secure the seat belt (with resistance set at one plate, rotate to an upright position and then tighten seat belt firmly).

3. Place your hands on your thighs (maintain a hand-thigh contact at all times during the exercise).

4. Lift-lower the weight with smooth, controlled movements.

What Are Some Basic Strength Training Exercises You Can Perform at Home?

If you are interested in starting a strength-training program, but not interested in joining a fitness center, you can perform a full-body workout at home. An effective workout can be completed with your own body weight or with minimal equipment, such as dumbbells, resistance bands, or tubing. The following exercises target all the major muscle groups and are designed to be performed in the convenience of your own home.

Lunge

Objective: To strengthen your hamstrings, quadriceps, and gluteal muscles.

1. Hold weights in your hands.
2. Step forward and bend your knees until in a lunge position.
3. Lower your trunk toward the floor by slowly bending at the knees to 90 degrees.
4. Return to the original position and repeat with your other leg.

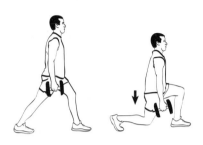

Standing Calf Raise

Objective: To strengthen the gastrocnemius.

1. Stand, using a chair for balance if needed.
2. Rise up onto the ball of your right foot through a full range of motion.
3. Return to the original position and repeat the required number of repetitions.
4. Repeat with the other leg.

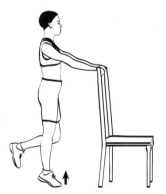

Modified Push-Up

Objective: To strengthen the pectoralis.

1. Begin on the floor by placing your hands slightly wider than shoulder width apart.
2. Push up, keeping your knees on the floor, extending to straight elbows.
3. Maintain a straight back.
4. Lower, so your upper arms are parallel with the floor, and repeat.

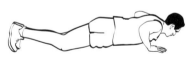

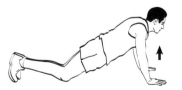

Bent Over Row

Objective: To strengthen the latissimus dorsi.

1. Slightly bend forward at the hips while maintaining a straight back.
2. Support your upper body with your other arm as shown.
3. Lift your arm up, raising the elbow to shoulder height.
4. Return to the starting position and repeat.

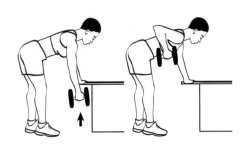

Lateral Raise

Objective: To strengthen the medial deltoid.

1. Stand with your feet shoulder width apart and knees slightly bent.
2. With your palms facing inward, lift your arms up and out to the side to shoulder level.
3. Lower the weight and repeat.

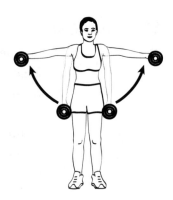

Triceps Kickback

Objective: To strengthen the triceps.

1. Flex at your hip (do not round out the back) leaning over the chair or table.
2. Raise your elbow so the upper arm is parallel with the floor and close to your body.
3. Use your other arm to maintain balance.
4. Start with the weight directly below the elbow.
5. Extend your arm at the elbow until the arm is straight.
6. Return to the starting position and repeat.

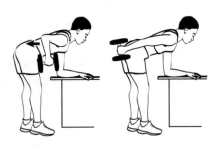

Standing Bicep Curl

Objective: To strengthen the biceps.

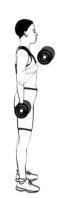

1. Keeping your upper arms close to your side, bend at the elbow, and raise the weight to your shoulders.

2. Return to a straight arm position and repeat.

3. Maintain your upper arm in the same position throughout the movement.

Prone Lower Back Extension

Objective: To strengthen the erector spinae.

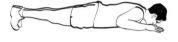

1. Lie face down, elbows bent, arms relaxed and resting on the floor.

2. Arch your back to a comfortable position and hold, keeping the arms relaxed throughout the movement.

3. Return to the starting position and repeat.

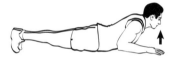

Abdominal Crunch

Objective: To strengthen the rectus abdominis.

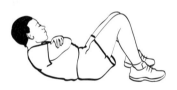

1. Lie on your back, knees bent, arms crossed over your chest.

2. Lift up your head and continue to lift your shoulders off the floor, toward your knees.

3. Keep your lower back in contact with the floor.

4. Return to the starting position slowly, maintaining the contraction, and repeat.

RUNNING AND WALKING TRAINING GADGETS—HOME STRENGTH TRAINING EQUIPMENT

To add more variety and challenge to your home strength training routine, consider purchasing exercise bands, tubes, balls, or dumbbells. There are several different models of each of these items on the market; the following are examples of some of the more commonly used brands. All descriptions taken directly from the products' websites.

Thera-Band® Resistance Bands (www.thera-band.com)—Bands are available in eight color-coded levels of resistance. Bands are lightweight, portable, and easy to store. Handles provide a secure grip to prevent injuries. Door anchors are also available for securing bands in a doorway to allow for a greater variety of exercises to be performed.

SPRI® Original Xertube (www.spriproducts.com)—Color-coded tubes provide varying levels of resistance. Handles at each end allow for a safe, effective workout. These tubes are lightweight, portable, and easy to store.

Resist-a-Ball® (www.resistaball.com)—This air-filled rubber ball can be used for many different upper-, lower-, and core body exercises. The ball not only helps you develop strength and endurance, it also helps to improve balance and posture. Resist-a-balls come in various sizes based on height.

Xerball® Medicine Balls (www.spriproducts.com)—These weighted balls help to improve strength, endurance, power, and stability. The balls can bounce allowing for unique exercises to be performed. Xerballs are extremely durable, maintaining their shape even after repetitive bounces.

Hampton Fitness Neo-Hex 3, 5, and 8 lbs. (www.hamptonfit.com)—These durable neoprene-coated dumbbells are safe on even hardwood floors. The multicolored weights come in 3, 5, and 8 lbs; a perfect set for a beginner.

How Can You Track Your Progress?

Keeping a log of your strength training is just as important as a log for your walking or running. Have your log in hand when performing exercises in the gym or at home in order to keep track of the sets, repetitions, and exercises completed. Your strength training program should be changed every four to eight weeks, and therefore a log also serves as a reminder of when to make adjustments to your regimen. Record your strength training in a notebook or on a formal log sheet (see Figure 8.3). In the appendix and on this book's website, you will also find an example of the Strength Training Log sheet. Keeping a log takes the guesswork out of your workout and helps you to stay motivated by showing you how much you have improved.

tip

Make sure you have your strength training log before heading to the gym so you can keep track of your progress.

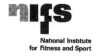

National Institute
for Fitness and Sport

Strength Training Log

NAME EXERCISE			DATE 4 / 21 / 05 WT/REPS	DATE _/_/_ WT/REPS	DATE _/_/_ WT/REPS	DATE _/_/_ WT/REPS	DATE _/_/_ WT/REPS	DATE _/_/_ WT/REPS
UPPER BODY	CHEST PRESS	1 2 3 4	15 / 12 15 / 12 15 / 10 __ / __	__ / __ __ / __ __ / __ __ / __	__ / __ __ / __ __ / __ __ / __	__ / __ __ / __ __ / __ __ / __	__ / __ __ / __ __ / __ __ / __	__ / __ __ / __ __ / __ __ / __
	PULLOVER	1 2 3 4	30 / 8 30 / 8 __ / __ __ / __	__ / __ __ / __ __ / __ __ / __	__ / __ __ / __ __ / __ __ / __	__ / __ __ / __ __ / __ __ / __	__ / __ __ / __ __ / __ __ / __	__ / __ __ / __ __ / __ __ / __
	ROWING	1 2 3 4	40 / 9 40 / 9 40 / 10 __ / __	__ / __ __ / __ __ / __ __ / __	__ / __ __ / __ __ / __ __ / __	__ / __ __ / __ __ / __ __ / __	__ / __ __ / __ __ / __ __ / __	__ / __ __ / __ __ / __ __ / __
	SHOULDER PRESS	1 2 3 4	10 / 10 10 / 11 10 / 12 __ / __	__ / __ __ / __ __ / __ __ / __	__ / __ __ / __ __ / __ __ / __	__ / __ __ / __ __ / __ __ / __	__ / __ __ / __ __ / __ __ / __	__ / __ __ / __ __ / __ __ / __
LOWER BODY	LEG PRESS	1 2 3 4	100 / 14 100 / 14 __ / __ __ / __	__ / __ __ / __ __ / __ __ / __	__ / __ __ / __ __ / __ __ / __	__ / __ __ / __ __ / __ __ / __	__ / __ __ / __ __ / __ __ / __	__ / __ __ / __ __ / __ __ / __
	LEG EXTENSION	1 2 3 4	20 / 15 20 / 16 20 / 16 __ / __	__ / __ __ / __ __ / __ __ / __	__ / __ __ / __ __ / __ __ / __	__ / __ __ / __ __ / __ __ / __	__ / __ __ / __ __ / __ __ / __	__ / __ __ / __ __ / __ __ / __
	LEG CURL	1 2 3 4	15 / 14 15 / 14 15 / 13 __ / __	__ / __ __ / __ __ / __ __ / __	__ / __ __ / __ __ / __ __ / __	__ / __ __ / __ __ / __ __ / __	__ / __ __ / __ __ / __ __ / __	__ / __ __ / __ __ / __ __ / __
	CALF RAISE	1 2 3 4	__ / 15 __ / 15 __ / 15 __ / __	__ / __ __ / __ __ / __ __ / __	__ / __ __ / __ __ / __ __ / __	__ / __ __ / __ __ / __ __ / __	__ / __ __ / __ __ / __ __ / __	__ / __ __ / __ __ / __ __ / __
ABDOMINALS / BACK	ABDOMINAL CRUNCHES	1 2 3 4	50 / 13 50 / 13 __ / __ __ / __	__ / __ __ / __ __ / __ __ / __	__ / __ __ / __ __ / __ __ / __	__ / __ __ / __ __ / __ __ / __	__ / __ __ / __ __ / __ __ / __	__ / __ __ / __ __ / __ __ / __
	BACK EXTENSION	1 2 3 4	50 / 11 50 / 12 __ / __ __ / __	__ / __ __ / __ __ / __ __ / __	__ / __ __ / __ __ / __ __ / __	__ / __ __ / __ __ / __ __ / __	__ / __ __ / __ __ / __ __ / __	__ / __ __ / __ __ / __ __ / __
		1 2 3 4	__ / __ __ / __ __ / __ __ / __	__ / __ __ / __ __ / __ __ / __	__ / __ __ / __ __ / __ __ / __	__ / __ __ / __ __ / __ __ / __	__ / __ __ / __ __ / __ __ / __	__ / __ __ / __ __ / __ __ / __
		1 2 3 4	__ / __ __ / __ __ / __ __ / __	__ / __ __ / __ __ / __ __ / __	__ / __ __ / __ __ / __ __ / __	__ / __ __ / __ __ / __ __ / __	__ / __ __ / __ __ / __ __ / __	__ / __ __ / __ __ / __ __ / __

FIGURE 8.3

Sample strength training log.

Do Yoga and Pilates Count As Strength Training?

Yes. Yoga and Pilates can provide a change of pace from the traditional strength training exercises. For both exercises, take a class or sign up for an individual session with a reputable, certified, and experienced instructor. Yoga and Pilates require knowledge of proper form and technique to ensure a safe and effective workout. Classes can be found in most fitness centers as well as private yoga or Pilates studios. Home videos are also available if you are interested in exercising at home.

How Can Yoga Improve Strength?

As mentioned earlier in this text, yoga was developed in India and has been evolving for about 5,000 years. Yoga exercises focus on the entire body, and involve a combination of stretching and strengthening postures, breathing exercises, and meditation. Muscular strength and endurance is gained by holding your body in specific positions for a short period of time. These static positions challenge the muscles through *isometric contractions* as well as controlled, flowing movements. Isometric means the exercise does not involve movement—you are holding the same position, requiring your muscles to support and stabilize your body. The flowing movements require strength and endurance to stabilize the body while moving through a range of motion in a smooth, controlled fashion.

How Can Pilates Improve Strength?

Joseph Pilates created what is now know simply as "Pilates." Joseph was an accomplished athlete and body builder who practiced yoga, boxing, and meditation. He developed a series of controlled, concentrated exercises that increase flexibility and focus on strength in the center (or core) of the body while also engaging the mind.

These flowing exercises are performed with quality, not quantity in mind. The power for the movements stem from the core of your body, which includes the abdominal muscles and lower back, and flows to the extremities. Most importantly, Pilates integrates the body as a complete unit during the exercise. Traditional strength training exercises often isolate muscles, working them individually. Pilates develops all of the muscles collectively, rather than separating them.

Pilates exercises are typically completed in one of two ways. The Pilates *matwork* is the most common form practiced today. The series of movements is performed while lying on a mat. Specialized equipment, such as the *Reformer*, can also be used with a trained Pilates instructor to perform the exercises.

What Are the Frequently Asked Questions Related to Strength Training?

This section will answer the most frequently asked questions by runners and walkers about strength training and dispel commonly held myths about the results of engaging in a regular strength training program.

Can muscular strength be maintained without training?

No. As with any other training modality, strength returns to pre-training levels if not maintained. Studies have shown that detraining does not occur as quickly in strength athletes as aerobic athletes, but without training consistently, strength will not be maintained.

What is required to maintain muscular strength?

As with cardiorespiratory training, one can maintain muscular fitness with fewer days per week than it took to acquire it. The key is that even though the number of training days is reduced, the intensity level increases slightly. Research has demonstrated that strength can be maintained on as little as one session per week when the lifts are completed with a minimum intensity of 75%–80% of one repetition maximum. However, very few individuals choose to lift with this level of intensity. It is best to lift according to ACSM's guidelines, reviewed earlier in this chapter.

I am female. Will weight training make me look less feminine? Will my muscles get the same size as a man's?

No. The inability of the average woman to develop large bulky muscles is normally attributed to low testosterone levels, the hormone required for building large amounts of muscle mass. The relatively large increase in strength experienced by women performing resistance training is accompanied by only a small increase in muscle mass and either a decreased or unchanged body weight. Any increase in muscle mass is typically balanced by a loss of adipose tissue.

Can muscle turn into fat and fat turn into muscle?

This is a common myth surrounding strength training. The truth is that muscle and fat are physiologically separate tissues. One can never "turn into" the other. Rather, when individuals stop training, their muscle mass will begin to atrophy due to disuse. Simultaneously, excess fat begins to accumulate because the individual is exercising less and probably eating the same or more than they were when they were strength training regularly.

Similar logic can be applied to the opposite scenario. When an individual begins a strength training program, muscle will begin to develop in the exercised areas. However, the muscle is not "replacing" fat tissue. Adipose tissue will begin to diminish simultaneously due to the calories burned during an exercise session and the rise in resting metabolic rate due to an increase in muscle mass. Fat loss can be maximized if strength training is combined with regular cardiorespiratory exercise and a well-balanced, calorie-appropriate diet.

Can I spot reduce?

No. People are genetically prone to storing fat in certain areas. Genetics is the main determinant on where weight is gained or lost. When fat is lost, as a result of expending more calories than consuming, it is lost from a variety of areas on the body. Although resistance training increases strength in the specific muscle group exercised, resistance exercise alone cannot eliminate fat from a specific area.

I am an avid runner. Will weight training make me bulky and decrease my running performance?

Studies have shown that a sport-specific weight training program will help improve running times and performance. Most elite athletes in a variety of sports incorporate some type of strength training in their weekly regimens. The key is developing an appropriate strength training program. A person primarily interested in running should not train like a bodybuilder or power lifter. Following the ACSM guidelines for strength training two to three days per week, performing 8 to 10 different exercises should be sufficient for a runner. The weight should be kept moderate and the repetitions within the 8–15 range. Done correctly, weight training can improve running performance. Do not worry about adding bulk with this type of weight training. Keep in mind that bulking up has a great deal to do with genetics (that is, amount of testosterone, skeletal frame size, muscle fiber type), diet, type of training, and amount of rest.

Will weight training decrease my flexibility?

It is a common misconception that weight training is responsible for decreasing flexibility. In actuality, lack of stretching and a failure to move through a full range of motion causes a decrease in flexibility. Many people who weight train extensively remain flexible because they practice going through a full range of motion and stretch daily.

THE ABSOLUTE MINIMUM

- Everyone can benefit from an appropriately planned strength training program.

- Strength training exercises should be performed at least two to three times per week.

- Integrate 8–10 different exercises into your routine, targeting the major muscle groups of the body.

- Perform at least one to two sets of 8–12 repetitions to volitional fatigue for each exercise.

- Traditional strength training exercises can be performed in a gym or at home.

- Non-traditional exercises, such as yoga and Pilates, can also be effective in increasing muscle strength and endurance.

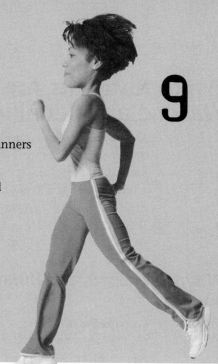

9

WHAT SHOULD YOU EAT TO FUEL YOUR WALKING AND RUNNING?

Consider nutrition training equal to physical training.

If you do not provide your car with the appropriate gas, it will not run efficiently. If you run out of gas, your car will stop. The same relationship holds true between your daily diet and your weekly walking and running. If you do not fuel your body properly, your training, as well as your health, will suffer. This chapter discusses the nutrients you need on a daily basis when training for a 5K, 10K, or half-marathon, how you can create healthy and quick meals, ideas for energy-packed recipes, and tips for dining out the healthy way.

Which Nutrients Are Important for Fueling Walking and Running?

As you progress through your training for a 5K, 10K, or half-marathon, you will be challenging your body on a regular basis through walking, running, cross training, strength training, and competitions. In order to keep up with the demands of the training, you need to adequately fuel your body on a daily basis with macronutrients (carbohydrate, protein, and fat) and micronutrients (vitamins and minerals). This section will review the purpose of the macro- and micronutrients and their relevance to walking and running.

Why Do Walkers and Runners Need Carbohydrates, Protein, and Fat?

Carbohydrates, protein, and fat are classified as *macronutrients* because they are required in large quantities on a daily basis by your body. Each macronutrient has a role in fueling running and walking as well as contributing to general health and well being. All macronutrients are classified as *essential* nutrients, indicating the need to consume them daily in sufficient quantities.

Carbohydrates are the main fuel for all types of physical activity, especially endurance sports such as walking and running. Carbohydrates are used by your muscles whether you are training for a 5K, 10K, or half-marathon. Without sufficient carbohydrates, your training sessions will feel more difficult, your pace will droop, and your recovery from workouts will be longer; therefore the importance of consuming adequate daily carbohydrates cannot be underestimated. Carbohydrates are also the main fuel for the brain and many other bodily processes that sustain your body daily. Due to the importance of carbohydrates for fueling the body, your total daily intake should be 50%–65% carbohydrates. Carbohydrates are found in a variety of foods including whole grains, fruits, vegetables, and dairy/dairy alternative products.

Proteins are involved in the development, growth, and repair of muscle and other bodily tissues. Protein can also be used for energy, however not efficiently, and therefore protein is not a preferred source of energy for your body. Although not a main source of fuel for walking and running, protein is critical for recovery for long, hard workouts. Therefore, protein should contribute 12%–20% of total daily calories. Proteins are found in a variety of foods including whole grains and vegetables, however mainly concentrated in the dairy/dairy alternative and meat/meat alternative groups.

Fats are primarily used as a fuel at rest and during low to moderate intensity exercise. Fats are also involved in providing structure to cell membranes, aiding in the production of hormones, lining of nerves for proper functioning, and facilitating the absorption of fat-soluble vitamins (vitamins A, D, E, and K). Fats have received much attention over the past couple of decades due to research linking dietary fats to an increased risk for chronic disease. Due to this link, dietary fats should be consumed in moderation, contributing 20%–30% of your total daily calories. Fats are concentrated in butter, margarines, salad dressings, and oils, but are also found in meats, dairy products, nuts, seeds, olives, avocados, and some grain products.

Ideally, every meal will consist of a carbohydrate, protein, and fat source to ensure you are consuming enough of each macronutrient throughout the day. In the next chapter, you will learn when it is important to eat each of these macronutrients before, during, and after walking and running.

Why Do Walkers and Runners Need Vitamins and Minerals?

Vitamins and minerals are classified as micronutrients because your body requires only small amounts of each nutrient every day. Similar to the macronutrients, vitamins and minerals are also considered essential and must be consumed regularly to prevent deficiencies. Vitamins and minerals are ideally obtained from the foods and beverages you eat throughout the day, with supplements taken sparingly and used only as extra insurance.

Vitamins do not directly provide energy to your body; however they aid in the extraction of energy from carbohydrates, protein, and fat. Vitamins are involved in a wide variety of bodily functions and processes that help to keep your body healthy and disease-free. Vitamins are classified as either water soluble (B-vitamins and vitamin C) or fat-soluble (vitamins A, D, E, and K). Vitamins are found in nearly all foods including fruits, vegetables, whole grains, meat/meat alternatives, dairy/dairy alternatives, and some fats. Refer to Figure 9.1 for the daily requirements (RDA), functions, and dietary sources of the water- and fat-soluble vitamins.

Minerals have a role in the structural development of tissues as well as the regulation of bodily processes. Physical activity places demands on your muscles and bones, increasing the need for oxygen-carrying compounds in the blood and increasing the loss of sweat and electrolytes from the body, which hinge on the adequate intake and replacement of dietary minerals. Minerals are categorized into major minerals (calcium, sodium, potassium, chloride, phosphorus, and magnesium) and trace minerals (iron, zinc, copper, selenium, chromium, and manganese) based on the total quantity required by the body on a daily basis. Similar to vitamins, minerals are found in a wide variety of foods, however, they are mainly concentrated in meat/meat alternatives and dairy/dairy alternatives groups. Refer to Figure 9.2 for the daily requirements (RDA), functions, and dietary sources of minerals.

FIGURE 9.1

Understanding vitamins.

NAME	RDA/AI*	FUNCTION	SOURCE
Vitamin A	700 ug (F) 900 ug (M)	Vision, growth, prevent drying of skin and eyes, promote resistance to infection	Liver, fortified milk, yams, spinach, carrots, apricots, cantaloupe, broccoli
Riboflavin	1.1 ug (F) 1.3 mg (M)	Essential for growth, energy metabolism	Milk, mushrooms, spinach, liver, enriched grains
Thiamin	1.1 mg (F) 1.2 mg (M)	Metabolism, nerve function	Sunflower seeds, lean meats, whole and enriched grains, peas
Niacin	14 mg (F) 16 mg (M)	Energy metabolism, fat synthesis and breakdown	Bran, fish, beef, chicken, peanuts, enriched grains
Folate	400 ug	DNA and RNA synthesis, amino acid synthesis, decrease risk of birth defects	Leafy greens, citrus fruits, whole and enriched grains, beans, orange juice, fortified cereals
Vitamin B6	1.3 mg 19-50yrs 1.5 mg (F > 50 yrs) 1.7 mg (M > 50 yrs)	Protein metabolism, hemoglobin synthesis	Animal protein foods, broccoli, bananas, beans, whole grains, citrus fruits
Vitamin B12	2.4 ug	Nerve function, red blood cell metabolism	Dairy products, chicken, pork, shellfish, beef
Vitamin C	75 mg (F) 90 mg (M) Add 35 mg for smokers	Collagen, hormone, and neurotransmitter synthesis, wound healing, iron absorption	Citrus fruits, strawberries, broccoli, greens, potatoes
Vitamin D	200 IU 19-50 yrs 400 IU 50-70 yrs 600 IU > 70 yrs	Facilitate absorption of calcium and phosphorous, maintain bone calcium	Fortfied milk, sardines, salmon, produced by body in response to sunlight
Vitamin E	15 mg	Antioxidant: prevent break-down of vitamin A and unsaturated fatty acids	Vegetable oils, wheat germ, peanuts, leafy greens, seeds
Vitamin K	90 ug (F) 120 ug (M)	Blood clotting	Leafy greens, broccoli, eggs, soybeans

(F) = Females   (M) = Males   IU = International Units   mg = Milligrams   ug = Micrograms   RDA - Recommended Dietary Allowances
AI - Adequate Intakes   *Amounts given for persons aged 19-70 unless otherwise noted.

FIGURE 9.2

Understanding minerals.

NAME	RDA/AI*	FUNCTION	SOURCE
Iron	18 mg (F) 19-50 yrs 8 mg (M) 8 mg (F) > 50yrs	Hemoglobin, immune function	Meats, leafy greens, seafood, dried fruits, beans, fortified cerals, nuts
Calcium	1000 mg 19-50 yrs 1200 mg > 50 yrs	Bone and teeth formation, transmission, muscle contraction	Dairy products, leafy greens, some tofu, canned fish with bones, fortified orange juice
Zinc	8 mg (F) 11 mg (M)	Enzyme function, wound healing, growth, immunity	Seafoods, meats, greens, beans, whole grains, eggs, poultry
Magnesium	310-320 mg (F) 400-420 mg (M)	Bones, nerve and heart function	Whole grains, legumes, tea, broccoli, nuts, beans, bananas, soy beans
Chromium	25 ug (F) 19 - 50 yrs 20 ug (F) > 50 yrs 35 ug (M) 19 - 50 yrs 30 ug (M) > 50 yrs	Metabolism of carbohydrates and fats	Whole grains, meat, cheese, egg yolk, fortified cereal, mushrooms
Sodium	≤ 1500 mg 19 - 50 yrs ≤ 1300 mg 50 - 70 yrs ≤ 1200 mg > 70 yrs	Electolyte and water balance, nerve transmission	Table salt, processed foods
Potassium	4700 mg	Electrolyte balance, nerve transmission	Bananas, meat, beans, orange juice, yogurt, potatoes
Phosphorous	700 mg	Bone and teeth formation, energy production	Dairy products, meat, fish, beans, sodas, eggs
Copper	900 ug	Aids in protein metabolism	Beans, nuts, whole grains, shellfish, dried fruits, cocoa
Selenium	55 ug	Antioxidant functions	Meats, fish, eggs, milk, seafood, whole grains
Manganese	1.8 mg (F) 2.3 mg (M)	Enzyme action including carbohydrate metabolism	Nuts, oats, beans, tea, rice, whole grains
Chloride	≤ 2300 mg 19 - 50 yrs ≤ 2000 mg 50 - 70 yrs ≤ 1800 mg > 70 yrs	Maintain fluid and acid-base balance	Table salt, processed foods, fish

(F) = Females   (M) = Males   mg = Milligrams   ug = Micrograms   RDA - Recommended Dietary Allowances
AI - Adequate Intakes   *Amounts given for persons aged 19-70 unless otherwise noted.

How Can You Incorporate Balance, Variety, and Moderation into Every Meal?

Because all nutrients play a role in supporting your walking and running, you need to focus on consuming these nutrients on a daily basis. You can achieve balance, variety, and moderation throughout the day by planning appropriate meals. This section will provide tips and hints to help you create healthy meals for you and your family. Keep in mind that "healthy" does not have to mean "tasteless" and "time-consuming." Healthy, energy-packed recipes that will excite your taste buds and rejuvenate your body for the next workout are presented later in this chapter.

Balance is the first key to meal-planning success. The best tip in this category is to aim for three different food groups in every meal. For example, if you had cereal with milk and a banana for breakfast you would have consumed three food groups (grains, dairy, and fruit). Ideally, every meal will have, at a minimum, one fruit or vegetable, a protein source (meat/alternative or dairy/alternative), and then one more food group to balance out the meal. If you strive for at least three food groups in every meal, the next two meal planning tips will be easier to put into practice.

Variety is a close partner with balance in regard to meal planning success. Although you may achieve the goal of three food groups at every meal, you may not master variety if you choose the same three foods for each meal every day. Variety pertains to food selections between and within each food group. All food groups (whole grains, fruits, vegetables, dairy/dairy alternatives, and meat/meat alternatives) should be represented in a healthy diet. Completely eliminating an entire food group increases your risk for developing a nutrient deficiency. However, deficiencies can also result from eating a limited variety of foods within each food group. For example, yogurt and cheese are excellent sources of calcium, which is essential for strong bones and teeth. However, yogurt and cheese do not contain vitamin D. Vitamin D is found primarily in fluid milk. If you are eating yogurt and cheese but avoiding milk, you may be consuming sufficient amounts of calcium, but putting yourself at risk for a vitamin D deficiency. Each food has a unique nutrition profile providing various nutrients. Aim for three food groups per meal *and* be creative with your meal planning to incorporate different foods every day.

The final consideration for healthy meal planning is *moderation*. Moderation is a foreign concept in the area of eating for most Americans. Moderation relates to appropriate portion sizes. The "typical" American portions are two to three times larger than the recommended serving sizes. Because of this consistent overconsumption of food, Americans are gaining weight every year. Although you will need more energy to fuel your walking and running, you need to continue to be cognizant of what is considered an appropriate serving and how many servings you need in a day. Table 9.1 in the next section reviews the recommended serving sizes for each food group and the number of servings from each group that would be appropriate for active runners and walkers.

Full meal plans for various calorie levels are presented later in this chapter to provide examples of how to achieve balance, variety, and moderation within one meal or snack as well as throughout the day.

How Many Servings from Each Food Group Should You Consume?

Table 9.1 outlines the recommended serving sizes for each food group and the number of servings an active runner or walker will need in a day for a proper training diet. The suggested ranges for the number of servings consumed per day may vary greatly. Consider the following factors to estimate if you should strive for the low end of each range or the high end of each range:

- *Age*—as you grow older, you will need fewer calories to sustain your energy levels and body weight. If you are 40 years old or younger, aim for the middle to high end of the ranges; if you are older than 40, aim for the middle to lower end of the spectrum.

- *Gender*—Men generally burn more calories than women, thus requiring more food throughout the day. The reason men burn more calories than women is mainly because men genetically have more muscle mass, our metabolically active tissue. In general, men should aim for the middle to high end of each range, while the women should strive for the middle to low end of each range.

- *Activity Level*—As your weekly mileage increases, your calorie expenditure and nutrient needs will also increase. If you are training for a half-marathon, aim for the middle to high end of the ranges; if your goal is to walk or run a 5K or 10K, aim for the middle to low end of the ranges.

Keep in mind that everyone is different and therefore your specific needs may be outside the ranges provided in the chart. Consult with a dietitian to determine exactly how many servings from each food group you need in a day to meet your needs.

tip

You can find a dietitian in your area by visiting the American Dietetic Association web site (www.eatright.org) and clicking on "Find a Dietitian."

Table 9.1 also provides the suggested number of servings from each food group for a pre-activity meal and a snack. Pre-activity meals should include at least three food groups; however, snacks typically include only one to two food groups. More information about establishing the best pre-activity meal for you will be discussed in the next chapter.

Table 9.1 Constructing a Healthy Training Diet for Walkers and Runners

Food Group and Serving Sizes	Training Diet	Pre-Activity Meal	Snack	Important Nutrients & Functions
Grains Bread, *1 slice* Cold cereal, *1 oz* Pancake, *1 (4 inch in diameter)* Rice, pasta, *1/2 cup* Cooked cereal, *1/2 cup* Muffin, roll, bagel, *1 medium*	6–12	2–3	1–2	Carbohydrates to supply energy to the muscles and brain; B-vitamins to help the body convert food to energy
Vegetables Chopped raw or cooked, *1/2 cup* Leafy raw vegetables, *1 cup*	3–5+	1	1–2	Carbohydrates to supply energy to the muscles and brain; vitamin A and beta carotene for healthy skin and eyes
Fruits Fresh, *1 medium piece* Canned fruit, *1/2 cup* Dried fruit, *1/4 cup* 100% juice, *3/4 cup*	2–4+	1–2	1–2	Vitamin C for healthy body tissues and aid in iron absorption; potassium for normal heart function and muscle contraction; water to prevent dehydration
Dairy/Dairy Alternatives Skim or 1% milk, *1 cup* Soy or rice milk, *1 cup* Low-fat yogurt, *1 cup* Low-fat cheese, *1–2 oz* Cottage cheese *1/4 cup*	3–4+	1	1	Protein for the growth and repair of muscle tissue as well as a healthy immune system; calcium, and vitamin D for healthy bones and teeth
Meat/Meat Alternatives Cooked beef, fish, poultry, *2–3 oz* Dried beans, peas, lentils, *1.5 cups* 1 egg or 2 Tbsp peanut butter counts as 1/3 of a serving	3–4	1	0–1	Protein for the growth and repair of muscle tissue as well as a healthy immune function; zinc for healthy immune function; B-vitamins to help the body convert food to energy; iron for healthy red blood cells to carry oxygen; fat for energy and essential fatty acids required by the body

What Are Examples of Meal Plans Based on Various Calorie Levels?

While training for an endurance running or walking event, it is imperative to eat a balanced diet containing the nutrients needed for optimal performance and recovery. As your mileage increases, so will your nutrient requirements. Examples of balanced meal plans are provided in the following pages, ranging from 15%–18% protein, 56%–62% carbohydrate, and 23%–26% fat.

The volume of food changes based on the amount of physical activity performed during the day. For example, a day of rest will demand fewer total calories than a 12-mile run or walk day! Remember, each person's calorie requirements will vary; therefore use these menus as guidelines and ideas of how to develop an adjustable, appropriate menu for you. For variety, the menus also include some of the delicious recipes (items in bold) provided within this chapter.

tip

Eat only until satisfied. Eat regularly throughout the day. If you are hungry between meals, snack on fruit, yogurt, granola bars, cheese and crackers, or trail mix.

Water is listed for some meals. However, water intake should be consistently maintained throughout the day.

1800 Calories (Rest Day)

Breakfast	1 cup Raisin Bran
	1/2 cup skim milk
	6 oz orange juice
Lunch	Pita sandwich:
	1/2 whole-wheat pita round
	2 Tbsp **spicy orange hummus**
	3 oz sliced ham
	1 slice Swiss cheese
	2 tomato slices
	1 leaf of lettuce
	3 slices of bell pepper
	(red, green, or yellow)
	1 cup of vegetable soup
	10 saltine crackers
	16 oz water

Snack	8 oz vanilla fat-free yogurt
	1 cup fresh strawberries
	1/4 cup granola
	16 oz water
Dinner	1 cup **tuna noodle casserole**
	1/2 cup grapes
	2 cups spinach leaves with
	1/2 tomato, chopped
	1 1/2 Tbsp chopped walnuts
	2 Tbsp olive oil/vinegar dressing
	8 oz skim milk

Menu Composition

	Total	Percent of Calories
Calories	1857	—
Protein	86 g	18%
Carbohydrate	271 g	56%
Fat	55 g	26%

2200 Calories (3–5 Mile Run/Walk Day)

Breakfast	8 oz skim milk
	3 1/2 inch plain bagel
	2 Tbsp peanut butter
	1 orange
Snack	1/2 cup pineapple chunks in its own juice
	1 **NIFS Bar**
Lunch	1 medium baked potato
	1 cup **veggie chili**
	2 Tbsp shredded cheddar cheese
	10 saltine crackers
	6 oz mixed berry yogurt
	16 oz water

Snack	1/2 cup trail mix (dried fruit, nuts, cereal)
	16 oz water
Dinner	**Spicy Turkey Burger** with a whole wheat bun and 1 slice Swiss cheese
	2 cups mixed salad with 1 Tbsp light dressing
	1 cup chopped cantaloupe

Menu Composition

	Total	Percent of Calories
Calories	2215	—
Protein	91 g	16%
Carbohydrate	339 g	59%
Fat	63 g	25%

3000 Calories (10–12 Mile Run/Walk Day)

Breakfast	1 cup oatmeal, dry with
	1 Tbsp honey
	1/2 cup skim milk
	3 Tbsp raisins
	1 Tbsp chopped nuts
	2 slices of toast
	1 1/2 tsp butter or margarine
	8 oz cranberry juice
Snack	1 granola bar
	1 apple
Lunch	Peanut butter & banana sandwich:
	2 slices whole wheat bread
	2 Tbsp peanut butter
	1 medium banana, sliced
	1 cup carrots
	1/2 cup fresh broccoli

1/3 cup **spicy orange hummus** as a dip for the vegetables

2 fig newtons

16 oz water

Snack

1 oz Colby-jack cheese

8 wheat crackers

16 oz water

Dinner

Stir fry:

    2 cups brown rice, cooked

    1 1/2 cup stir-fried vegetables

    2 Tbsp coarsely chopped nuts

    1/4 cup pineapple tidbits, drained

    3 oz steamed shrimp

5 steamed asparagus spears

2 Tbsp cheese sauce

Menu Composition

	Total	Percent of Calories
Calories	3037	—
Protein	118 g	15%
Carbohydrate	487 g	62%
Fat	81 g	23%

What Are Examples of Healthy, Energy-Packed Recipes?

Now that you are balancing work, school, family, training, and other commitments, you need quick, easy recipes to fix on the fly. In addition to making your meals in minutes, the recipes you choose should also supply your body with the proper nutrition to keep you going strong all day long. The following recipes fit these criteria—

tip

Drink plenty of water throughout the day. During training for a 5K, 10K, or half-marathon, your fluid needs can range from 64–100+ oz per day!

quick, easy, *and* healthy. Some of the following recipes are included in the meal plans presented in this chapter. Enjoy!

NIFS Bar

24 dried dates	1/4 tsp baking powder
1/3 cup honey	1 Tbsp canola oil
4 Tbsp orange juice	1/4 cup maple syrup
2 Tbsp lemon juice	2 egg whites
2 1/2 cups whole wheat flour	1 tsp lemon juice
1/2 tsp baking soda	

Combine dates, honey, orange juice, and 2 tablespoons lemon juice into a food processor and chop. In a mixing bowl, combine the wheat flour, baking soda, baking powder, canola oil, maple syrup, egg whites, and one teaspoon lemon juice. Beat with an electric mixer three to four minutes at medium speed. Add the date mixture and beat until blended. Spray an 8"×11" baking dish with cooking spray and spread the dough evenly. Bake at 350°F for 10 minutes or until they are warm and a bit puffy. Refrigerate to harden. Makes 12 bars.

Nutrient Analysis per Serving

Calories: 192 calories	Protein: 4.4 g
Carbohydrates: 43 g	Fat: 1.7 g
Fiber: 4.3 g	Iron: 1.3 g
Calcium: 21 mg	Vitamin C: 3.4 mg

Chocolate Banana Smoothie

1 banana	1 to 2 Tbsp cocoa powder
1 cup skim or soy milk	1/2 to 1 cup ice cubes
1/2 cup plain yogurt	

Place all ingredients in a blender and mix until smooth. Makes 1 serving.

Nutrient Analysis per Serving

Calories: 262 calories	Protein: 17 g
Carbohydrates: 49 g	Fat: 1 g
Fiber: 3 g	Iron: 1 mg
Calcium: 548 mg	Vitamin C: 13 mg

Spicy Orange Hummus

1 15-oz can chickpeas (garbanzo beans)

1 Tbsp bean juice from the chickpea can

1/4 cup orange juice

2 Tbsp rice vinegar

2 tsp lite tamari (organic soy sauce)

1 tsp Dijon mustard

1/4 tsp ground turmeric

1/4 tsp ground cumin

1/4 tsp paprika

1/4 tsp ground ginger

1/4 tsp ground coriander

1/4 cup dried parsley leaves

Place all ingredients in a food processor. Blend until smooth. Serve with cut vegetables, whole wheat pita bread, or use as a sandwich spread. Makes 5 servings.

Nutrient Analysis per Serving

Calories: 95 calories

Carbohydrates: 15 g

Fiber: 3.5 g

Calcium: 36 mg

Protein: 4 g

Fat: 2 g

Iron: 1.7 g

Vitamin C: 10 mg

Super Juice

1 cup juice (orange, pineapple, or your favorite juice)

1 cup water

1/8 tsp salt

Combine all ingredients and shake. Can be used as an alternative to sports beverages. Makes 1 16-oz serving.

Nutrient Analysis per Serving

Calories : 112 calories

Carbohydrates: 27 g

Fiber: 0.5 g

Calcium: 27 mg

Protein: 0 g

Fat: 0 g

Iron: 0 mg

Vitamin C: 97 mg

Veggie Chili

1 28-oz can diced tomatoes

2 15-oz cans pinto beans, drained

1 15-oz can red kidney beans, drained

1 15-oz can garbanzo beans, drained

1 14.5-oz can hominy, drained

2 cups water

1 6-oz can tomato paste

1 4-oz can chopped green chilies

2 medium onions, chopped

2 medium zucchini, sliced

2 medium carrots, sliced

3 Tbsp chili powder

1 tsp ground cumin

3/4 tsp garlic powder

1/2 tsp sugar

1 cup shredded Monterey Jack cheese

Combine all ingredients except cheese in a Dutch oven. Bring to a boil and then reduce heat. Cover and simmer for 30 minutes. Serve hot with 1 Tbsp of shredded cheese on top. Makes 12 (2 cup) servings.

Nutrient Analysis per Serving

Calories : 240 calories

Carbohydrates: 40 g

Fiber: 11 g

Calcium: 164 mg

Protein: 12 g

Fat: 5 g

Iron: 3 g

Vitamin C: 30 mg

Tuna Noodle Casserole

1 Tbsp olive oil

1/2 red pepper, chopped

1 medium onion, chopped

1 cup mushrooms, sliced

1 1/2 cups frozen mixed vegetables

1/4 cup whole wheat flour

2 1/2 cups skim milk

1 12-oz package pasta shells, cooked according to package directions

1 1/2 cups shredded Monterey jack cheese, divided

2 9-oz cans tuna, packed in water

1 Tbsp dried parsley

1/2 tsp salt

1/2 tsp black pepper

1/3 cup Parmesan bread crumbs

Preheat oven to 350°F. Spray 13×9-inch baking dish with non-fat cooking spray. Set aside. Pour olive oil into a large skillet at medium heat. When hot, add pepper, onion, mushrooms and mixed vegetables. Sauté 5 minutes or until cooked and tender. In a medium bowl, whisk flour and milk together until smooth. Stir into vegetable mixture and cook 5 minutes or until thickened, stirring constantly. Remove skillet from heat. Stir in cooked pasta. Add 1 cup of cheese and stir until melted. Stir in tuna, parsley, salt, and pepper. Pour mixture into baking dish. Bake 25 minutes. Sprinkle last 1/2 cup of cheese and breadcrumbs over casserole. Bake 5 minutes or until cheese is melted and crumbs are golden. Makes 12 servings.

Nutrient Analysis per Serving

Calories : 205 calories	Protein: 18 g
Carbohydrates: 17 g	Fat: 7 g
Fiber: 1.8 g	Iron: 1.4 g
Calcium: 183 mg	Vitamin C: 13 mg

Spicy Turkey Burger

1 lb ground, lean turkey	1 cup sliced mushrooms
2 tsp garlic powder	cooking spray
1 tsp Cajun seasoning	4 whole wheat hamburger buns
1/4 tsp black pepper	8 slices tomato
1 medium onion, sliced	4 lettuce leaves

Combine first 4 ingredients. Divide the mixture into 4 equal portions, shaping each into a patty. Using a non-stick skillet on medium heat, add cooking spray. When the skillet is hot, add onions and mushrooms. Cover skillet and cook 10 minutes until vegetables are golden, stirring frequently. Remove vegetables from the pan; keep warm. Add cooking spray to the skillet. Place patties in the pan; cook 5 minutes on each side. Continue cooking to desired doneness. Compile burger, topping each patty with onion/mushroom mixture, 2 tomato slices, and a piece of lettuce. Makes 4 burgers.

Nutrient Analysis per Serving

Calories : 341 calories	Protein: 27 g
Carbohydrates: 33 g	Fat: 12 g
Fiber: 5.4 g	Iron: 4 g
Calcium: 72 mg	Vitamin C: 12 mg

Spinach Lasagna

1 lb ricotta cheese

1 1/2 cup shredded mozzarella
cheese

1 egg

10 ounces frozen chopped spinach
(thawed and drained)

1 tsp salt

1/2 tsp pepper

1/2 tsp oregano

32 oz of spaghetti sauce

12 oz uncooked lasagna noodles

1 cup water

In large bowl, mix ricotta, 1 cup mozzarella, egg, spinach, salt, pepper, and oregano. In greased 13×9-inch pan, layer 1/2 cup of sauce, 1/3 of the noodles, and half of the cheese mixture; repeat. Top with remaining noodles, and then remaining sauce. Sprinkle with remaining cheese. Pour water around edges. Cover tightly with foil. Bake at 350°F for 1 hour and 15 minutes. Let stand 15 minutes before serving. Makes 12 servings.

Nutrient Analysis per Serving

Calories : 189 calories

Carbohydrates: 21 g

Fiber: 4 g

Calcium: 305 mg

Protein: 14 g

Fat: 5 g

Iron: 6 mg

Vitamin C: 15 mg

Is It Possible to Dine Out and Eat Healthy?

Americans have more than doubled their food dollars spent outside of the home since 1955. With our busy lives, we are turning to dining out instead of spending time cooking at home. Sometimes it can seem challenging to find healthy options when dining out. However, by asking questions and using a few basic tools, you can put together restaurant meals that will fuel your body properly for running and walking with options that are low in fat and high in fiber, vitamins, minerals, and other nutrients.

Eating healthy when dining out involves asking the right questions, searching the menu for creative substitutions, and altering your behaviors. Use the following tips when dining out:

- Order first; you will tend to be less influenced by what others order.
- Eat slowly and engage in more conversation.
- Ask for sauces, salad dressings, and other condiments on the side.
- Remember that alcohol can increase your appetite and provides added calories without added nutrients.

■ Be selective when eating from a salad bar—choose fruits, vegetables, and low-fat dressings versus croutons, bacon, cheese, and full-fat dressing.

■ Remove tortilla chips or breadsticks from the table if you feel tempted to eat more than you should.

■ Eat a portion of the meal and take the remaining home in a doggie bag.

■ If your food does not come the way you ordered it, send it back!

What Should You Look for on the Menu?

Restaurants use descriptive adjectives on menus to describe the way foods are prepared. The following descriptions can help you determine whether a low-fat preparation or high-fat preparation technique was used for a particular food item:

Look for Low-Fat Preparation	Instead of High-Fat Preparation
Steamed; roasted; in its own juice; poached; garden fresh; broiled; tomato sauce; baked; marinara sauce	Au gratin; creamed; basted/braised; crispy; fried/pan-fried; buttered; casserole; sautéed; cheese sauce; gravy; escalloped; hollandaise

To choose healthy, lower fat, higher nutrient-dense options to fuel your body for walking and running, review the following list outlining items to choose "more often" and "less often" within the categories of beverages, salads, bread, potatoes and starches, vegetables, and entrees. When dining out, search the menu for the items in the "more often" categories and order the items in the "less often" categories only infrequently.

Beverages

Choose more often:

Water, juice, low fat milk, coffee, unsweetened iced tea

Choose less often:

Whole milk, milkshakes, regular soft drinks, alcohol

Salads

Choose more often:

Tossed green salad with vegetable toppings, fat free or vinegar dressing, fresh fruit salad, grilled chicken salad, salads with a small amount of nuts

Choose less often:

Potato salad, coleslaw, taco shell salads, regular dressing, olives, cheese, eggs, croutons, Caesar salad

Bread

Choose more often:

Plain breads, rolls, bread sticks, French bread, bagels

Choose less often

Sweet rolls, muffins, biscuits, croissants, doughnuts

Potatoes and Starches

Choose more often:

Baked, boiled, or mashed potatoes, corn, rice, pasta (without cream/butter sauces)

Choose less often:

French fries, au gratin, scalloped, or hash browned potatoes, potatoes with sauces or gravies

Vegetables

Choose more often:

Boiled, baked, or steamed vegetables

Choose less often:

Fried, au gratin or creamed vegetables, vegetables with sauces or gravies

Entrees

Choose more often:

Baked, roasted, or broiled: fish, poultry, lean beef, veal, lamb, pork; pasta with marinara sauce; pizza with vegetable toppings

Choose less often

Fried or breaded meats, casseroles, meats with gravy or sauces, pasta with white or cream sauces, eggs, sausage, bacon, quiche, hash

note

If you do choose an item high in calories or fat from the "choose less often" section, eat a small portion and compliment it with a healthier food item.

Should You Ask for Menu Substitutions?

Do not be afraid to ask questions of your server to gain clarification on menu items or to inquire about substitutions. By asking politely, you will be surprised at how accommodating most restaurants will be! The following questions will help you find or create the healthiest options on the menu:

- How is the food prepared?
- Do you have a light or healthy menu?
- Do you have low-fat salad dressing or sauces?
- May I have the toppings on the side?
- Can you leave off the sauce or gravy?
- Can I have it prepared without salt?
- Can I substitute a salad or fresh fruit for the French fries?

The Bottom Line: Dine Out Less and Eat In More

Although healthy choices can be made at most establishments, preparing meals at home is ideal. Cooking your own foods, specific to your individual needs, will be the best way to ensure you are getting the nutrition you need to train for a 5K, 10K, or half-marathon. Aim to decrease the number of times per week you dine out and when you do, search the menu for the healthiest options.

before you head out the door

Pack a lunch and snacks for a day at school or at work. By having foods available, you are less likely to be tempted to dine out for lunch or visit the vending machines midday.

RUNNING AND WALKING TRAINING GADGETS—COOKBOOKS AND DINING OUT GUIDES

Information is often the best tool when learning how to make healthy food and beverage choices. Cookbooks are an excellent resource for new ideas for quick, healthy, and tasty meals and snacks. The nutrition information provided by restaurants or in review books can reveal hidden calories and fat in menu items, thus making healthier options easier to distinguish. The following are only two of many books available to walkers, runners, and individuals who cook and dine out frequently. All descriptions taken directly from the products' websites.

The New York City Marathon Cookbook (http://web1.nyrrc.org/books.htm#b6) by Nancy Clark, M.S., R.D. (Rutledge Hill Press, 1994)—*The New York City Marathon Cookbook* is a valuable resource filled with quick-and-easy food suggestions. It reveals the tricks to eating a healthful, hassle-free sports diet—the kind of diet eaten by marathon champions and other athletes who prefer to spend their time training rather than cooking. The recipes are made from common foods, easy to prepare, and perfect for single people and families alike.

Restaurant Confidential (www.amazon.com) by Michael F. Jacobson, Ph.D. and Jayne G. Hurley, RD. (Workman Publishing, 2002)—*Restaurant Confidential* is a survival guide to eating out. It reveals the calories, sodium, and fat in close to 1,000 foods. The book reviews a majority of ethnic restaurant options, fast food establishments, and other foods commonly found at the movies or in the mall.

THE ABSOLUTE MINIMUM

- Include a combination of carbohydrates, protein, and fat in your daily diet, with an emphasis on the master fuel for running and walking—carbohydrates.

- Strive to consume your daily requirements of vitamins and minerals from a variety of food sources throughout the day.

- Aim for three food groups in every meal. Snacks should include one or two different food groups.

- The key components to healthy meal planning for active runners and walkers are balance, variety, and moderation.

- Learn what counts as a serving and eat an appropriate number of servings from each food group per day.

- Try new recipes!

- Dine out in a healthy way by asking questions of your server, searching the menu for creative substitutions, and altering your ordering and eating behaviors.

- The best foods and fluids to consume before running and walking

- The amount and type of fluid to drink while running and walking

- When and how to use sports drinks, bars, and gels

- The optimal post-activity meal or snack

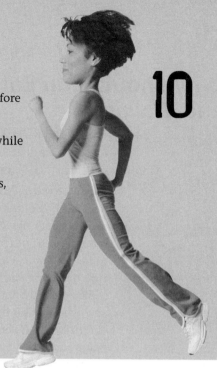

10

TRAINING AND COMPETITION NUTRITION FOR RUNNERS AND WALKERS

Nutrition can make or break your race.

Training sessions will seem easier and muscles will feel fresh and energized when you eat appropriately before, during, and after running and walking. On the other hand, you can feel tired, bloated, and sore if you don't fuel appropriately. For race day, a well-planned and executed nutrition strategy will allow you to feel and perform at your best; a haphazard nutrition plan can cause all of your hard work during training to go down the drain.

Why Should You Eat Before Running and Walking?

Many runners and walkers ask "Do I need to eat anything before running and walking?" The answer is definitely yes. There are several reasons why you should fuel up with a meal or snack before heading out the door:

■ *To provide energy, preventing a decrease in blood sugar at the start of a walk or run.* Our bodies need energy for endurance exercise. When you eat before you exercise, your blood sugar will be within the normal range at the start of your run or walk. For those of you training for a 5K or 10K, a meal or snack before your training session should be sufficient to keep your energy level high throughout your workout. However, if you are training for a half-marathon, you need to consume a sports beverage and/or other carbohydrate-rich products during training, in addition to your pre-activity meal or snack, to keep energy levels sustained during the long walks and runs.

> **tip**
>
> If your blood sugar begins to drop, your body will start slowing down and you may not be able to finish your planned walk or run. If your blood sugar drops significantly, you will begin to feel light-headed, nauseated, and weak.

■ *To ward off feelings of hunger or weakness.* If you are hungry at the start of a walk or run, it can be a distraction from focusing on proper form, the intensity of your session, or just relaxing!

■ *To provide a psychological edge and feeling of well-being.* By fueling up before walking and running, you will feel better mentally, giving you the mental boost to continue going strong. The mental component becomes increasingly important as the distance or duration of your walk or run increases. For those of you training for a half-marathon, eating before you head out the door is a must!

What Kind of Foods Should You Eat Before Training or Racing?

Now that you know it is imperative to eat before running and walking, the next question to answer is "What should you eat?" When planning a pre-activity meal or snack consider the following guidelines:

▪ *High in complex carbohydrates.* Carbohydrate-rich foods are easily digested and provide the best source of energy for the body. Carbohydrates are the preferred source of energy for working muscles and therefore essential for optimal performance in any physical activity. Foods such as pasta, rice, whole-grain breads, cereals, fruits, and vegetables are good selections. Do not cut yourself short in this area!

▪ *Moderate in protein.* Protein is primarily important for maintaining and building muscle tissue. However, it also has several roles for endurance sports. Because it slows digestion slightly, protein helps to sustain energy levels for longer periods of time. Secondly, a portion of the energy needed to run and walk is derived from protein, albeit a small portion. Therefore, small to moderate amounts of protein-rich foods are important to consume before exercising. Pre-activity protein sources should be low-fat, such as two to three ounces of lean meat, poultry, or fish; boiled or poached eggs; skim or one percent milk; one ounce of low-fat cheese or cottage cheese; or soy products.

▪ *Low in fat.* Fat (that which is stored in our body) is an important energy source, especially for endurance events. High fat foods, however, are not the best choices for a pre-activity meal because they slow digestion. It is best to avoid foods like chips, fried foods, sausage and other prepared meats, mayonnaise-type sandwich spreads, and regular salad dressings in the pre-activity meal.

▪ *Low in refined sugars.* Refined sugars are a source of carbohydrate that are found in foods such as candy, soda pop, cookies, cakes, pies, honey, and table sugar. Even though these foods provide carbohydrates, they are not ideal choices before running and walking. Negative side effects of eating sugary foods right before exercise can include stomach upset, diarrhea, and hypoglycemia (low blood sugar), all of which can have a negative effect on running and walking. Refined sugars also do not have any "staying power," which causes your energy to peak quickly but does not last for any length of time.

▪ *Focus on familiar foods.* Be sure to eat foods that are tried and true before heading out the door to walk or run. You want to make sure that what you eat does not cause an upset stomach or other gastrointestinal distress while exercising. Test several different meals before running and walking during your training to determine the "ideal" meal for race day.

▪ *Adequate amounts of fluids.* Fluids can be obtained in the form of water, juice, or milk. Drink at least two to three cups of fluids two to three hours prior to exercise, and then an additional one cup of fluid 10–20 minutes before exercise.

When Should You Eat Before Training or Racing?

Eating and drinking nutritious, energy-packed foods and fluids will lead to a great run or walk, but only if consumed at the appropriate time. When planning your pre-activity meal, consider the following factors, which will affect the timing of your meal:

- High calorie meals take longer to leave the stomach than smaller snacks.
- The more intense the activity, the more digestion time is needed.
- High fiber foods (specifically beans and legumes) may slow digestion. These foods are great to include in a daily diet, but may not be best for consumption immediately before running or walking. If you do choose to include these foods, allow more time for digestion.
- Liquid meals are digested quickly and easily.

Taking the above points into consideration, in general allow for the following digestion times:

- Three to four hours for a large meal.
- Two to three hours for a smaller meal.
- One to two hours for a light snack, blended, or liquid meal.
- Less than an hour for a small snack, depending on your tolerance.

Keep in mind that the terms "large," "small," and "light" are all relative terms. For example, what you might consider a "light snack" may in fact be a "large meal" to a training partner. You need to determine which meals are considered "large" or "small" and the digestion time you need before you feel comfortable enough to run or walk. The following is a sample menu for a low-fat, high-carbohydrate meal that could be eaten about two to three hours before a workout or competition.

Two slices whole grain bread

Two to three ounces of sliced turkey

One to two servings of fruit

One cup skim or 1% milk

Mustard or low-fat mayonnaise if desired

Water

before you head out the door

Do not walk or run on an empty tank of gas. Eat or drink something—ranging from a glass of juice to a pancake breakfast—before heading out the door.

HEALTHY PRE-ACTIVITY MEALS AND SNACKS

Here are some more ideas for healthy, pre-activity meals or snacks:

Cereal with skim milk and banana

Poached egg on dry toast

Pancakes with syrup

Peaches with low-fat cottage cheese

Low or non-fat yogurt with applesauce and cinnamon

Pasta with tomato sauce

Cheese and veggie pizza, thick crust

Vegetable soup with crackers

Yogurt and fruit blended in the blender

A NOTE FOR RACE DAY

A case of nerves before a big event can make it difficult to eat. If this happens to you, be sure to eat well the day before. Have a substantial dinner and a bedtime snack. If there is a "magic or special" food for you, be sure to pack it when traveling to an event. Carbohydrate foods that travel well include dried fruits, bagels, fig bars, animal crackers, bread sticks, and apples and oranges just to name a few. Always eat familiar foods before competition. Save the new stuff for training. New foods increase the risk of an upset stomach, cramping, and heartburn, which may decrease performance in your planned race.

Why Should You Focus on Fluids?

Oftentimes, runners and walkers are diligent about their weekly mileage, purchasing new shoes in a timely fashion and registering for races months in advance. However, most people don't think twice about their hydration status. Drinking fluids on a regular basis and staying well-hydrated is not only important for your ability to meet your running and walking goals, but it is also critical for health and safety. Read this section closely!

What Function Does Fluid Have in Your Body?

Fluid (mainly water) is needed by all body cells. It regulates body temperature, carries nutrients and oxygen to cells, removes waste, lubricates all joints, and protects organs and tissues. Our bodies are actually about 67 percent water.

During activity, adequate fluid intake is essential to prevent dehydration and maintain optimal performance. Not only can dehydration negatively affect athletic performance, but it also can lead to serious conditions such as heat exhaustion or even heat stroke. (For a reminder of the signs, symptoms, and treatment of heat exhaustion and heat stroke see "Recognizing and Treating Heat Exhaustion and Heat Stroke" in Chapter 4, "Safety Precautions.") In this chapter you will determine how much fluid to drink before and after running and walking, as well as the amount you need to drink during running and walking (because everyone is different). It is imperative that you understand and implement proper hydration guidelines to prevent dehydration, or the more serious hyponatremia.

What Is Hyponatremia?

In recent years, the incidence of a condition called hyponatremia has become more prevalent in runners and walkers. *Hyponatremia* is a disorder of fluid-electrolyte balance that results in abnormally low sodium concentrations in the blood. If sustained, hyponatremia can lead to a variety of neurological dysfunctions which, left untreated, can escalate into seizures, coma, or death. The signs and symptoms of hyponatremia include headache, nausea, dizziness, vomiting, or seizures. Hyponatremia is an issue mainly for those of you running or walking a half-marathon. For those who are focusing on shorter distances, you are generally not at risk for hyponatremia, but knowledge and prevention is important for everyone.

Hyponatremia can be caused by a variety of factors including

- Consuming too much fluid prior to training or an event.
- Drinking fluid in excess of individual sweat losses.
- Drinking only water (versus sports beverages) during endurance exercise (longer than one or two hours).
- Running or walking for more than four hours.
- Taking NSAIDs (non-steroidal anti-inflammatory drugs), such as Advil® or Aleve® before or during exercise. NSAIDs cause the body to increase its excretion of sodium.

By drinking appropriate amounts and types of fluid before, during, and after running or walking, you can effectively prevent both dehydration and hyponatremia.

How Much Should You Drink Before, During, and After Running and Walking?

Drink plenty of cool fluids before, during, and after a workout or competition. In general, allow your body's thirst mechanism to drive your drinking. However, be aware that it is possible to lose up to two quarts of sweat before becoming noticeably thirsty! Therefore, you need to drink regularly. On the other hand, as mentioned previously, if you drink too much you could be putting yourself at risk for hyponatremia. By following established guidelines, and determining your individual sweat rate, you can strike a balance between these two extremes.

The following recommendations, published by the National Athletic Trainers' Association in 2000, will help you maintain hydration and optimize athletic performance:

- *Drink at least 8–12 cups of fluid each day* (1 cup = 8 ounces). Juices, milk, coffee, tea, water, and other beverages all count towards your daily total.

- *Drink two to three cups of fluid, two to three hours before exercising.* This quantity of fluid will allow you to be well hydrated at the start of a run or walk, without causing you to visit the bathroom multiple times before or during your workout.

- *Drink 1 cup of water 10–20 minutes before the workout.* The purpose of this big gulp of fluid is to top off your fluid tank before exercising.

- *Drink at least 1 cup (8 ounces) of fluid every 10–20 minutes during exercise* (24–48 ounces per hour). This guideline is one of the hardest for runners and walkers to put into practice. Many people drink only small amounts during exercise (less than 16 ounces per hour) or nothing at all! If you aren't currently in the habit of drinking while running and walking, start consuming small amounts, and then progress gradually toward your individual "optimal" amount based on your sweat rate. The steps to determine your sweat rate will be presented in the next section.

After an exercise session, drink two to three cups for every pound of body weight you lose during exercise. Part of the upcoming calculation of your individual sweat rate is weighing before and after a run or walk. Any weight lost during one workout is attributed to fluid loss (not fat loss). For every pound you lose during one exercise session, you need to consume two to three cups (16–24 ounces) of fluid. Once you establish your

caution

You should not gain weight during an exercise session. If you do, know that you are drinking too much fluid. Perform a sweat trial to more accurately estimate your needs.

individual sweat rate and drink accordingly, the amount of weight you lose in one workout should be minimal. Another way to know whether you have replaced all the fluids lost during activity is to monitor the color and frequency of urination. When your urine is a pale color and you are urinating about once every one or two hours, you can be confident that you are adequately hydrated.

How Do You Determine Your Individual Sweat Rate?

Each person sweats at a different rate. You must be aware of your typical sweat loss patterns to accurately calculate your specific fluid needs during exercise. For most people, 24–48 ounces per hour during exercise is appropriate for replacing lost fluids. The procedure of determining your sweat rate is accomplished by performing a *sweat trial*. Perform several sweat trials in different external environments—that is, various temperatures and relative humidity—to establish a drinking plan for any condition. Fluid needs will increase as the temperature and humidity levels rise and vice versa for cooler, less humid days.

caution

Do not underestimate the importance of determining your individual sweat rate! This is a critical calculation for keeping healthy and strong.

You can calculate your fluid needs per hour during running or walking by following these "sweat trial" steps:

1. Measure your body weight before exercise.
2. Record the length of your exercise session (in hours) and the quantity of fluid consumed.
3. Measure your body weight after exercise without sweaty clothes, and before using the restroom.
4. For every pound of body weight lost during exercise, an additional 16–24 ounces of fluid should have been consumed during that exercise session in order to stay well hydrated.
5. Add the quantity of fluid consumed during your run or walk (from step 2) to the fluid equivalent (based on weight loss during exercise from step 4), and divide that number by the total hours engaged in activity.

For example, Susie goes out for a six-mile walk that takes two hours to complete, drinking 24 ounces during her walk. She weighed 145 pounds before her walk and 143 pounds afterward. Following the steps stated here, she calculated her fluid needs as follows:

1. Weight before exercise = 145 pounds
2. Length of exercise = 2 hours of walking

   Quantity of fluid consumed = 24 ounces
3. Weight after exercise = 143 pounds
4. Weight loss during activity = 145 – 143 = 2 pounds

   Fluid equivalent = 2 lbs. × 16–24 ounces = 32–48 ounces of additional fluid needed
5. Fluid consumed during exercise = 24 ounces

   Fluid equivalent based on weight lost = 32–48 ounces

   24 ounces + 32–48 ounces = 56–72 ounces

   Divide 56–72 ounces by 2 hours = 28–36 ounces per hour

Therefore, Susie should aim to consume 28–36 ounces of fluid per hour during future walks under the same environmental conditions.

What about those of you training for shorter distances that last less than an hour? You will follow the same process as set out previously. Just make sure that you convert minutes into hours for the last step. For example, Dave is training for his first 5K running race. He has progressed to running 2 miles at a 10-minute/mile pace, making his longest run 20 minutes. He performed a sweat trial and discovered that he lost 0.5 pound (175 pounds before and 174.5 pounds after) in his 20 minute run. He forgot his water bottle at home and therefore did not drink anything during his run. To complete his sweat trial calculation, Dave would take the following steps:

1. Weight before exercise: 175 pounds
2. Length of exercise: 20 minutes of running

   Quantity of fluid consumed: 0 ounces
3. Weight after exercise: 174.5 pounds
4. Weight loss during activity: 175 – 174.5 = 0.5 lbs

   Fluid equivalent: 0.5 lbs. × 16–24 ounces = 8–12 ounces of additional fluid needed
5. Fluid consumed during exercise: 0 ounces

   Fluid equivalent based on weight lost: 8–12 ounces

   0 ounces + 8–12 ounces = 8–12 ounces

   Divide 8–12 ounces by 0.33 hours (20 minutes ÷ 60 minutes = 0.33 hours) = 24–36 ounces per hour

By knowing his fluid losses per hour, Dave can calculate his fluid needs for any run that lasts less than an hour. In this example, he could simply use the information obtained through his weight loss to determine his fluid needs for another 20-minute run because he did not consume any fluid. However, once he progresses to a 30- or 40-minute run, it will be handy to know his fluid needs per hour. He can use the 24–36 ounces of fluid per hour as a standard, and then divide that number by the length of his run. For anything less than an hour, Dave needs to determine the percentage of an hour he will run, and then multiple that percentage by 24–36 ounces. A 30-minute run would require 12–18 ounces ($30 \div 60 = 0.5 \times 24$–36 ounces = 12–18 ounces in 30 minutes); a 40-minute run would require 16–24 ounces ($40 \div 60 = 0.66 \times 24$–36 ounces = 16–24 ounces in 40 minutes).

You will need to perform several sweat trials, establish a drinking plan, and then practice your plan in a majority, if not all of your runs and walks. Through practice, your body will become trained to tolerate fluids, ultimately making your race experience comfortable and memorable.

Now That You Know How Much to Drink...What Should You Drink?

The quantity of fluid you need is only one part of the ultimate hydration equation. You also need to learn what type of fluid will be best for you to consume. There are many beverages on the market that target runners and walkers: plain water, juices, sports beverages, energy drinks, fitness waters, oxygenated waters, and so on. The type of fluid best for you will depend on several factors; however, the main determinant is the length of your running and walking sessions.

Cool water is almost always a good choice. It is easy to obtain, inexpensive, and absorbed relatively quickly. However, once the length of your runs and walks extend beyond 60–90 minutes, you should switch to sports beverages.

In long training sessions and competitive events, a sports drink is the preferred beverage because it supplies water, carbohydrates, and electrolytes. Because carbohydrates are the main fuel for working muscles, consuming a source of carbohydrates during running and walking will increase your endurance and keep you energized. Electrolytes, mainly sodium and potassium, are lost in sweat. They need to be replaced during exercise that lasts longer than 60–90 minutes to prevent conditions such as hyponatremia. Look for a sports drink that has about 50–80 calories, 14–19 grams of carbohydrates, and 100–165 milligrams of sodium per 8 ounces. Be aware that many of the "fitness" waters do not have sufficient amounts of carbohydrates and/or electrolytes and therefore are not the best choice for long distance running and walking.

Beverages that contain caffeine and alcohol are not good choices. Caffeine and alcohol are diuretics, which contribute to fluid loss and dehydration. Read the labels of "energy drinks" carefully. Many of these products contain large doses of caffeine and refined sugars in high concentrations.

Fruit juices are great choices for the training diet and after a workout or competition. They are not, however, a good choice during running and walking. Drinking juices after a workout will help replace fluids, carbohydrate to refuel the muscles, and electrolytes lost through sweat. However, because of their high carbohydrate concentration, they may cause stomach cramping and diarrhea if consumed during exercise.

before you head out the door

Weigh yourself before heading out the door to begin gathering the information for your sweat trial calculation. Once you have established your sweat rate, be sure to take a bottle filled with the appropriate amount of either water or a sports drink, based on the length of your walk or run.

RUNNING AND WALKING TRAINING GADGETS—WATER BOTTLES

In order to have fluids easily accessible during running and walking, a water bottle is an essential piece of training gear. There are several different models of water bottles: hand-held bottles, waist-belt bottle holders, and backpack fluid containers. The following list describes several examples of these products on the market. All descriptions taken directly from the products' websites.

Hand Held Bottle Gripper (www.nathansports.com)—The gripper fastens onto a 20–24 oz. bottle to transfer the weight of the bottle, thereby relieving the strain on your fingers. The strap is adjustable to fit any size hand. Each gripper has a small pocket for money, keys, or identification.

REI Quick Shot Waistpack (www.rei.com)—A waist belt features a single 20 oz bottle holder in a molded-foam packet. It includes a zipper pocket for holding keys or money.

The Fuel Belt (www.fuelbelt.com)—This waist belt has a design featuring an even distribution of bottles. The Endurance model holds a total of 28 ounces in four small bottles. It allows for the runner or walker to carry several different types of drinks—different flavors of sports drinks or water.

CamelBak CATALYST™ (www.camelbak.com)—Waistpack design allows for a "hands-free" method of carrying fluid. This lightweight and stable model makes carrying your liquids comfortable for both runners and walkers. It holds 0.8 liter (27 ounces), allowing for longer training sessions with minimal refilling.

Which Sport Supplements Are Appropriate During a Run or Walk?

In today's multi-billion dollar world of sports, performance foods are becoming increasingly popular. Athletes of all kinds are looking for ways to increase their stamina, prevent fatigue, and give themselves the extra edge to succeed. To supply this demand, manufacturers have invented a variety of performance foods for runners and walkers, consisting of sports drinks, energy bars, and energy gels. These products are designed primarily to provide quick fuel to the working athlete, but also to be digested easily, convenient to carry while running and walking, and nonperishable. Most of the following products can be purchased at local grocery stores, sports and athletic stores, and often at fitness centers.

Are Sports Drinks Necessary During Running and Walking?

Sports drinks are a mixture of water, carbohydrates, and electrolytes (potassium and sodium). In general, sports drinks are most beneficial when the duration of a workout or competition exceeds one hour. However, some research has also shown benefits for activities that last less than one hour. In one hour or more of continuous running or walking, a sports drink can supply carbohydrates for working muscles as well as fluid and electrolytes that are lost through sweat. This will allow the body to perform at a more optimal level for a longer period of time.

Sports drinks are considered a better choice for hydration during activity than fruit juices and soft drinks because they contain a lower concentration of carbohydrates. Juices and soft drinks typically contain 10%–11% sugar solution, whereas sports drinks contain approximately 6%–8% sugar solution. Fluids with a high concentration of carbohydrates (for example, juices and soft drinks) are absorbed by the stomach much slower than sports drinks and can cause gastrointestinal distress. The 6%–8% sugar solution in sports drinks allows for fast absorption, as well as energy. Look for sports drinks containing 6%–8% carbohydrates (14–19 grams of carbohydrate per 8 ounces of the beverage) and 100–200 milligrams of sodium per 8 ounces of fluid.

See Table 10.1 for a comparison of commonly used sports drinks.

Table 10.1 Comparison of Commonly Used Sports Drinks

Sport Drink	Calories	Carbohydrate (CHO) %	CHO	Protein	Fat	Sodium
Gatorade	50	6%	14 g	0 g	0 g	110 mg
Gatorade Endurance	60	6%	15 g	0 g	0 g	200 mg
Powerade	70	8%	19 g	0 g	0 g	53 mg

Table 10.1 (continued)

Sport Drink	Calories	Carbohydrate (CHO) %	CHO	Protein	Fat	Sodium
All Sport	70	8-9%	19 g	0 g	0 g	55 mg
Accelerade	79	6%	14 g	3 g	0 g	125 mg
Cytomax	48	7%	10 g	0 g	0 g	70 mg

What Are Energy Bars and When Should You Use Them?

Today's energy bars can be divided into two categories: bars that are high in carbohydrates and low in protein and fat, and those that are high in protein and low in carbohydrates and fat. Each type of bar serves a different purpose. Bars high in carbohydrates and low in fat and protein are beneficial to consume before or during running or walking. Consume the high-carbohydrate bars at least 30–60 minutes before a walk or run, or eat small portions of the bar throughout a long workout that lasts more than one hour. Walkers typically find the bars easier to digest while moving than runners. Bars high in protein and low in carbohydrate and fat are appropriate for a mid-day snack, when taken several hours prior to a workout, or immediately following a workout. Drink at least 12–16 ounces of water during and after the consumption of any bar.

See Table 10.2 for a comparison of commonly used energy bars.

Table 10.2 A Comparison of Commonly Used Energy Bars

Energy Bar	Bar Type	Calories	Carbohydrates	Protein	Fat
Power Bar	High Carb*	230	45 g	10 g	2.5 g
Bolder Bar	High Carb	210	40 g	8 g	3 g
Clif Bar	High Carb	230	42 g	10 g	4 g
Luna Bar	High Carb	180	26 g	10 g	3 g
MET-Rx	High Carb/Pro†	340	50 g	27 g	2.5-4 g
Steel Pro Bar	High Pro+	330	15 g	30 g	6 g
Balance Bar	High Pro	200	22 g	14 g	6 g
Pure Protein Bar	High Pro	280	9 g	33 g	7 g
ProteinPlus Bar	High Pro	290	38 g	24 g	5 g

* High carbohydrate bars contain 55% or more of their total calories from carbohydrates.

† High carbohydrate/high protein bars meet both of the conditions listed here for carbohydrates and protein.

+ High protein bars contain 25% or more of their total calories from protein.

What Are Energy Gels and When Should You Use Them?

Energy gels consist mainly of carbohydrates (maltodextrin and polysacchrides). The carbohydrates in gels break down quickly into glucose to provide fast fuel for the body. Most energy gels range between 80–120 calories with 20–30 grams of carbohydrates and are generally fat and protein free. Energy gels are most beneficial to endurance athletes such as walkers and runners because they are convenient to carry, fast and easy to consume, and provide a source of energy during a long workout. Gels are not recommended as a snack before or after activity; instead they should generally be consumed during a workout or competition that lasts longer than 60–90 minutes. Consume at least eight ounces of water with every gel.

See Table 10.3 for a comparison of commonly used energy gels.

before you head out the door

If you are going to be walking or running longer than 60–90 minutes, fill your bottle with a sports drink and pack an energy bar or gel to take with you.

Table 10.3   A Comparison of Commonly Used Energy Gels

Performance Gels	Calories	Carbohydrates	Protein	Fat
Power Gel	110	28 g	0 g	0 g
Carb-BOOM	110	27 g	0 g	0 g
ClifShot	100	23 g	0 g	0.5 g
Hammer Gel	91	23 g	0 g	0 g
GU	100	25 g	0 g	0 g

What Are the Best Foods to Eat After Running and Walking?

Foods consumed after a walk or run can affect how you feel the next day, or even the next week. The foods chosen for a post-activity meal or snack are as important as those chosen before walking and running. Wise post-activity food choices facilitate a quicker and more complete recovery of the muscles' energy stores by allowing the muscles to rebuild and repair, thus preparing them for the next workout. A general guideline is to consume a 200–300 calorie snack within 30 minutes of a run/walk. The snack, as well as your subsequent well-balanced meal, should contain fluids, carbohydrates, protein, and electrolytes.

What Fluids Should You Drink After Running and Walking?

One of the top priorities after exercise is to replace the fluids lost during exercise due to sweating. The most appropriate fluid choices for after a workout include: water (plain and simple), fruit juices (which supply water), carbohydrates, and electrolytes. Watery foods such as fruits, vegetables, and soups also supply water, carbohydrates, electrolytes, and a variety of vitamins/minerals.

As stated earlier, drink 16–24 ounces of fluid for every pound of body weight lost during a run or walk. Complete rehydration, especially after runs or walks lasting longer than 60–90 minutes, can take 24 to 48 hours or more; therefore, drink an appropriate amount after exercising, and then continue to drink fluids throughout the rest of the day.

Why Are Carbohydrates Important After Running and Walking?

Carbohydrate-rich foods and beverages should be consumed as soon as possible following your run or walk. Carbohydrates will replenish your glycogen stores (the body's carbohydrate reserve) so you will feel refreshed and energetic for your next run or walk. The goal is to eat at least a half a gram of carbohydrate per pound of body weight within the first hour post-exercise. For example, an individual weighing 150 pounds would require 75 grams of carbohydrates. Ideally, this quantity of carbohydrate would be supplied in a balanced meal eaten after a run or walk. However, if it will be several hours before your next planned meal, have a small snack that contains the appropriate amount of carbohydrates, and then eat again at your normal mealtime. Using the example of a 150-pound person, the following snacks are good choices, each containing about 75 grams of carbohydrate:

- One cup orange juice and a small bagel
- One bowl of cereal, banana, and skim milk
- One cup low-fat fruited yogurt and four graham cracker squares
- Two ounces dried fruit and two ounces of pretzels

Why Is Protein Important After Running and Walking?

Amino acids (the building blocks of dietary proteins) are needed to help stimulate protein synthesis to repair tissues after exercise. Running and walking, especially the long distances required for half-marathon training, cause micro-tears in the muscle tissue. This muscle damage necessitates a little protein boost to kick-start the rebuilding process. Aim to consume 15–25 grams of protein within 30–60 minutes after a workout, as well as a complete meal that contains a good protein source within two hours.

Examples of high quality protein sources to eat after running and walking include the following:

- Lean meats (such as chicken, turkey, or fish)
- Low-fat dairy products (such as milk or yogurt)
- Legumes, nuts, and seeds
- Soy products (such as soy milk, tofu, or tempeh)

Why Are Electrolytes Important After Running and Walking?

In addition to water, relatively small amounts of sodium and potassium (electrolytes) are lost in sweat. With the exception of individuals in ultra-endurance events (lasting more than four to eight hours), these losses are easily replaced with the foods and fluids consumed on a daily basis. During a two-hour workout, it is possible to lose 180 milligrams of potassium and 1,000 milligrams of sodium. One medium banana contains 500 milligrams of potassium and one ounce of pretzels about 400 milligrams of sodium. Other nutrient-dense and sodium-rich options for after exercise include vegetables juices, soups, or cheese and crackers. At races, most of these foods may not be available; instead, look for sports drinks and salty snacks to munch on until you can have a well-balanced meal.

THE ABSOLUTE MINIMUM

- Eat within three to four hours of running and walking. You will need to eat more for longer runs or walks and less for shorter distances.
- Stay well hydrated at all times. Perform a sweat trial and drink accordingly during exercise.
- Use performance foods appropriately. Sports drinks are essential for any run or walk that is greater than 60 minutes. Energy bars and gels are needed only during runs and walks that last longer than 60–90 minutes.
- Eat a 200–300 calorie snack immediately following a run or walk. Focus on fluids, carbohydrates, protein, and electrolytes for a quick and complete recovery from running or walking.

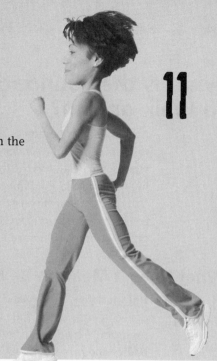

11

MENTAL TRAINING AND MOTIVATION

Maintain your motivation by shifting your mindset.

Americans have become quite proficient at starting an exercise or diet program, but fail miserably at maintaining an established, long-term regimen. To reap the benefits of physical activity and exercise, you must move your body on a regular basis for the rest of your life. Although this may seem daunting or near impossible, you can make this a reality by shifting your mindset about movement. This chapter will provide you with many different concepts and tools to help you incorporate physical activity into your daily routine forever.

What Is the Foundation of Your Motivation to Walk or Run?

An important question to ask yourself is, "Why do I want to walk or run a 5K, 10K, or half-marathon?" Understanding the source of your driving force to exercise provides some insight to the longevity of your physical activity habits. A book written by Jay Kimiecik, *The Intrinsic Exerciser*, explains how to shift your mindset from exercising because of extrinsic motivating factors to intrinsic factors. By focusing on your intrinsic reasons for exercising, you can greatly increase the likelihood that you will be a walker or runner for life.

What Does It Mean to Be Motivated by Extrinsic Factors?

Unfortunately, many Americans are not regularly active and for those who are active, a large percentage will quit exercising within several months of initiating a program. Why does this happen? Don't people realize how good exercise is for their bodies and minds? In fact, yes, most people recognize the long-term health benefits of exercising regularly. However, exercising solely for the anticipated physical and mental benefits is a perfect example of being motivated by extrinsic factors.

Extrinsic motivation is derived from outside sources. Oftentimes individuals begin an exercise program because of a doctor's recommendation, prodding from a friend or family member, or just because they feel like they "should." Although there is no doubt that engaging in an exercise program will improve physical/mental health and energy levels, exercise is not meant to be "work," a "chore," or "torture." If you are slugging through your walks and runs merely because you know you are supposed to exercise, you need to shift your mindset to be successful long-term.

Accordingly to Jay Kimiecik, if you do not find an *inner* reason to exercise, you will not continue exercising for a lifetime. The next section explores ways to find your intrinsic motivation for moving.

> **note**
>
> "Thirty minutes out, and something lifts...the fatigue goes away and feelings of power begin...after the run...I'm back to life with long and smooth energy, a quiet feeling of strength...the most delicious part is the night's sleep." –Mandell

What Does It Mean to Be Motivated by Intrinsic Factors?

Adults have forgotten how to play. Our time is spent only on functions that will produce a result—activities merely for the enjoyment of the activity are often considered a waste of time. This is especially true in the area of exercise. Adults often exercise because they "have to" or only because of the desired physical results of exercise. When you are motivated intrinsically, you will exercise because you *want to* move, not because you *have to* move. In the book *The Intrinsic Exerciser*, Jay Kimiecik challenges you to shift your mindset about exercise through an understanding of four components to intrinsic motivation: vision, mastery, flow, and "inergy."

Vision involves visualizing yourself exercising and imagining how it will feel to move your body. This tool is especially useful when approaching race day. If you visualize yourself completing each mile of the 5K, 10K, or half-marathon, you are much more likely to be successful on race day. However, this tool can be used every day; visualize yourself walking or running after work, enjoying the fresh air, feeling your muscles working, and savoring the relaxing effects of exercise.

Mastery is your desire to improve and grow. Mastery for walking and running may be your desire to successfully complete each long walk or run during your training for your first 5K, 10K, or half-marathon. After you finish your race, mastery can also be implemented when you decide to walk or run another 5K, 10K, or half-marathon to improve your time or to challenge yourself with a race of greater length. The focus for improvement and growth should be centered on your goals and performance (intrinsic focus). Mastery does not support setting goals for improvement based on trying to achieve the performance levels of others (extrinsic focus). Practice this technique when setting short-term and long-term goals—it is all about you!

Flow is achieved when you are totally absorbed in the experience of your exercise session. Your goal is to "exercise in the moment" by concentrating on how the movement of your body feels during exercise as well as your surrounding environment, while releasing the thoughts and stress of the day. This technique doubles as an excellent stress management tool—give yourself a mental break from daily challenges, allowing your mind and body to relax and regain strength. You will know you have mastered this component when you finish a walk or run and you can say, "I was enjoying my walk/run so much that I lost track of time."

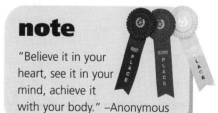

note

"Believe it in your heart, see it in your mind, achieve it with your body." –Anonymous

"Inergy" involves recognizing that the mind, body, and spirit are connected and that exercise can positively influence all three. Most people realize that

physical activity is a means to a healthier body; however, many do not consider the additional mental and spiritual benefits that result from physical activity. Regular exercisers often describe themselves as more alive, vibrant, energetic, relaxed, and grounded than when they were inactive. From a spiritual sense, many people engage in outdoor activities to connect with nature or their higher being. Start thinking about how you feel during and after your walks and runs to determine how exercise connects your mind, body, and spirit.

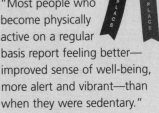

note

"Most people who become physically active on a regular basis report feeling better— improved sense of well-being, more alert and vibrant—than when they were sedentary." –Liz Applegate, Ph.D., R.D.

What Are Some Specific Motivational Tips to Keep You Moving in the Right Direction?

While working on your mindset shift from an extrinsic to an intrinsic focus on exercise, there are other ways you can motivate yourself on a daily basis. In this section, you will find a variety of specific suggestions on motivation to keep you walking and running during your 5K, 10K, and half-marathon training...and beyond.

How Can You Be Motivated by Setting Goals?

By setting goals, you establish a purpose for your training. If you have a reason for walking or running, you are more likely to stick to your exercise schedule. For example, by setting the goal to walk or run a 5K, 10K, or half-marathon, you have established a purpose for walking or running three to five times per week for 8–15 weeks. To stay motivated through goal setting, consider the following:

- *Set specific, realistic, and measurable goals.* Set goals that are challenging but within your reach, allowing you to improve while also enjoying the satisfaction of success.

- *Remember the tortoise and the hare.* Slow and steady progress toward your goals will get you to the finish line happy, healthy, and eager for more.

- *Keep records of your progress.* Success breeds success—document it, review it, and celebrate it.

- *Share your goal with others.* Tell someone your goal or post it someplace as a frequent reminder of your objectives.

RUNNING AND WALKING TRAINING GADGETS—EXERCISE AND NUTRITION LOGS

Don't forget the exercise, nutrition, and strength training logs in the appendix of this book that you can download in PDF form from this book's web page and print out for your use. (You can find this book's web page by navigating to http://www.quepublishing.com/ and typing the ISBN, 0789733145, into the Search field.) Recording your progress and reviewing your weekly success can be a great source of motivation and encouragement to continue walking and running.

How Can You Be Motivated by Your Program Design?

One of the most basic, as well as important, factors in keeping you motivated is your actual exercise routine or program design. When establishing your exercise regimen, consider the following tips:

- *Enjoy what you are doing.* If you don't enjoy your weekly activities, you will not continue long-term. Try different forms of exercise, especially on your cross training days, to find something fun and enjoyable!

- *Establish a routine you can follow on a weekly basis.* In this book, the protocols provide a daily and weekly plan to help you establish a routine to follow throughout your training for a 5K, 10K, or half-marathon.

- *Choose activities that fit your lifestyle and schedule.* Walking and running are excellent exercise options because they can be performed nearly anywhere, anytime. When deciding on cross training options, consider the activities that will fit most easily into your lifestyle and weekly schedule. Choose options that are nearby and convenient to make it easy to stick to your plan.

- *Add variety, the spice of life.* Incorporating several different modes of exercise into your weekly regimen will keep it exciting and fun. All of the protocols in this book schedule at least one day of cross training to allow you to discover and experience other physical activity options.

- *Avoid injuries through prevention.* Too much, too hard, too soon can lead to discomfort, long recovery periods after exercise, and ultimately an athletic injury. Start conservatively, progress gradually, take rest days, eat right, and stretch regularly to avoid any injury-related setbacks.

- *Find new routes to walk and run.* Explore your city to find new places to walk and run. A change of scenery can be invigorating!

How Can You Be Motivated by Making Time to Exercise?

One of the most common reasons people give for not exercising is a lack of time. However, it is actually not a *lack of time* but the *mismanagement* of time that prevents people from exercising regularly. Ensure you have time to exercise by considering the following:

- *Make an appointment with yourself to exercise.* Write it in your daily calendar and consider it just as important as your other meetings/appointments.

- *Exercise in the morning to avoid interruptions and delays.* As our days progress, there are more opportunities for challenges to arise that may prevent us from exercising. By planning to walk or run in the mornings, you can avoid unexpected interruptions or delays.

- *Maintain a habit of "mini" workouts when you are limited on time.* On your hectic days, remember that some exercise is better than no exercise. Therefore, even if you only have 10–15 minutes available in your day, make it productive by moving your body. Every minute counts!

- *Pack your exercise bag the night before a walk or run.* Plan ahead and pack your exercise bag with everything you need to successfully complete a walk, run, or cross training session (such as shoes, clothes, water bottle, post-workout snack, and so on).

- *When traveling, choose hotels with fitness centers.* Many hotels have fully equipped fitness centers or have associations with local health clubs. Shop around for the hotel that will allow you to stick to your exercise routine.

How Can You Be Motivated by the Buddy System?

Many people find that they are more motivated to exercise when they can share the experience with a friend or family member. If you prefer to make walking or running a social engagement, consider the following:

- *Find a committed partner and make use of the buddy system.* Committed is the key word—partner with someone who is as dedicated as you are so that you can support and encourage one another.

- *Involve your family.* By exercising together as a family, you become an excellent role model for your children by encouraging them to make physical activity a permanent part of their lifestyle.

- *Look into the programs offered by local health clubs.* If you are looking to meet new people who share similar goals, check out the activity programs at local fitness clubs and health centers. Many clubs offer structured training programs or encourage casual group meetings for people who are training for endurance events.

■ *Buy a large, fast dog that wants to walk you twice a day.* If you have ever thought about owning a pet, a dog can be an eager training partner.

How Can You Be Motivated by Your Attitude?

The mind is a powerful thing. If you have a negative attitude toward exercise, it will not be enjoyable and you will most likely not achieve your goals. However, with a positive attitude the possibilities are endless! Examine your attitude and then consider the following:

■ *Think positive.* Believe in what you are doing and know that you can reach your goals.

■ *Take control of your attitude and actions.* Realize that you have the power of choice in your everyday activities and exercise this power.

■ *You can change your attitude at any time.* Your attitude on a daily basis is largely defined by your perceptions and reactions to your daily environment. Oftentimes, you cannot change your environment, but you can change your thoughts and feelings related to a situation. Alter your perceptions and reactions in order to make a positive change to your attitude.

before you head out the door

Clear your mind and allow yourself to get absorbed in the experience of your walk or run. Choose to have a positive attitude and have fun.

How Can You Be Motivated by Rewards?

When you set a goal, you should also set a reward for achieving that goal. Consider choosing one of the following healthy rewards when you have accomplished a short or long-term goal:

■ Walking or running shoes

■ Walking or running apparel

■ A night on the town

■ Sports massage

caution

Avoid using food as your reward for achieving health and fitness goals as it can lead to an unhealthy relationship with food.

■ Magazine subscription

■ Sports nutrition book

■ Any other non-food item that will inspire you to continue exercising.

How Can You Overcome Some of the Common Roadblocks to Happiness?

Motivation to walk or run can be quickly squelched by our own mental traps. Too often walkers and runners compare themselves to others, strive for training perfection, or set unrealistic expectations that can create mental barriers to exercise satisfaction. When individuals get caught in one of these traps, the enjoyment of movement and overall training motivation declines, preventing the attainment of established goals. Don't let this happen to you! Read this section to learn how you can escape these mental traps.

How Can You Avoid the Comparison Trap?

In today's society, it is common for individuals to compare their performance to someone else's performance. However, constantly comparing yourself to others will lead you to focus on other's achievements while neglecting to acknowledge your own strides and accomplishments.

Keep in mind that all runners and walkers are not created equal. Someone will always be faster or run/walk further than you do. Do not fall into the comparison trap. Every person is unique, giving each of us the chance to enjoy running or walking for our own personal satisfaction. Learn to enjoy your accomplishments and celebrate them!

Set your goals, make your plan, and stick to it. Once you have accomplished a goal, celebrate it to recognize all the hard work you put into your training. By focusing on your goals and challenging yourself to improve for your unique reasons, you will realize the great satisfaction and happiness that accompanies hard work and dedication.

note

"It does not matter where I finish or how fast I run. Being a winner means doing my best." –George Sheehan

How Can You Avoid the Perfection Trap?

"Perfection belongs to the imaginary world," Thomas Moore wrote in his book *Care of the Soul*. Trying to run or walk perfectly in every training session or striving to have a "perfect" race can be mental roadblocks to fully enjoying the experience of successfully completing a 5K, 10K, or half-marathon.

Every workout or race will have its own hills, weather conditions, and mental challenges. These less than ideal conditions give the sport its character. It is the fulfillment of overcoming the challenges that makes success so sweet. Learning to appreciate the difficult days as well as the rewarding ones will make your training less stressful and more enjoyable. So, give up the perfection myth and enjoy the everyday challenges that running and walking offer.

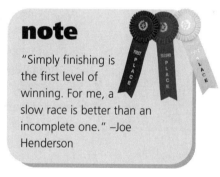

note

"Success in life is a matter not so much of talent as of concentration and perseverance." —C.W. Wendte

How Can You Avoid the Expectation Trap?

When you decide to run or walk a 5K, 10K, or half-marathon, you added the "runner" or "walker" title to your self-image. This addition to your image can also lead to increased expectations. Expectations that exceed your abilities can take the enjoyment out of training. Rather than enjoying what you have accomplished, you start dwelling on what you have not done. Dwelling on what you have failed to accomplish can add unnecessary stress to your training.

This does not mean that you should abandon your goals. Set small goals and focus on each one individually. Proceed toward your ultimate goal in small steps, taking pride in each accomplishment. Celebrating what you have achieved rather than dwelling on what you have yet to accomplish will make training much more enjoyable.

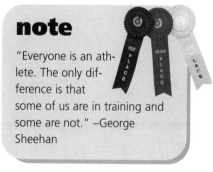

note

"Simply finishing is the first level of winning. For me, a slow race is better than an incomplete one." –Joe Henderson

note

"Everyone is an athlete. The only difference is that some of us are in training and some are not." –George Sheehan

What Can You Do to Stay Motivated?

Everyone is motivated in a different way. Take a minute to review this chapter and identify the concepts and/or suggestions that resonate with you. Then, document what you can do to stay motivated to exercise:

_____

_____

_____

_____

_____

THE ABSOLUTE MINIMUM

- Discover your intrinsic motivation to exercise in order to be successful long-term.

- Enjoy and celebrate the movement of your body.

- Motivate yourself by setting goals, following an exercise program that fits your needs, scheduling time to exercise, finding an exercise buddy, choosing a positive attitude, and rewarding yourself in a healthy way.

- Avoid common roadblocks to happiness by focusing on your goals, enjoying the challenge of long distance walking and running, and celebrating your accomplishments.

- Have fun!

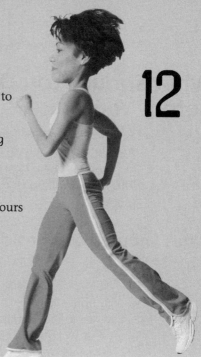

12

RACING STRATEGIES

It's show time!

You have trained hard for several weeks or months and you should feel confident that physically you are well prepared. However, this does not mean you can throw caution to the wind in the last week before your race. Your nutrition and fitness routine, sleep patterns, and mental preparation can make or break your race in the last couple of days or hours before you hit the start line. Read this chapter carefully—there are lots of small tips that can make a huge impact on your race experience and the successful attainment of your goal.

What Should You Do to Prepare in the Last Week Before Your Race?

You have worked hard during your training and you must be excited about your race! In order to stay calm and ensure the successful completion of your 5K, 10K, or half-marathon, there are a couple more things on your training "to-do" list. This section will provide a checklist of items to complete in the week leading up to race day.

What Should You Consider a Week Before Your Race?

Be sure to do the following a week before race day:

- *Check out parking options or drop off sites for race day arrival.* Anticipate heavy traffic the morning of a race. Think about where you want to park, how to get to that parking location, and the extra time that you might need in the case of a traffic jam. The last thing you need on race morning is the stress of delays and road rage!

- *Drive the course and be aware of hills, uneven pavement, shade, and other conditions.* By driving the course, you can develop a mental image of yourself successfully completing each section. The course review will also give you a huge advantage over others who are not aware of "hazards" along the course.

- *Note landmarks and where you can place your cheering section.* Do not underestimate the power of a support crew! A group of cheering fans can provide a huge boost when your physical or mental energy starts running low.

- *Know the finish—location, distance from last few turns, chute set-up, and so on.* By the time you get near the finish, you will not want to take any extra steps. Avoid going off course by knowing the full race course, including the finish line. At the finish line you will enter into a chute that will lead you across the actual line; dependent on the event, there may be different chutes for males, females, race distance, and so on. Remembering the landmarks close to the finish line will also give you mental boost knowing you are nearing the successful completion of your race.

- *Perform a mental rehearsal of the race.* Anticipate obstacles (such as untied shoes, cramps, stitches, falling down, and so on) and know how you will react to them so that when they occur you can respond and move on.

What Should You Consider Two Days Before Your Race?

Two days before the race, be sure to do the following:

- *A good night's sleep is important.* Most people are too excited or nervous the night before a race to sleep soundly. Therefore, plan on sleeping long and well two days before the race.

- *Start loading up on fluids and carbohydrates.* Refer to Chapter 10, "Training and Competition Nutrition for Runners and Walkers," for the appropriate pre-activity nutrition and fluid guidelines. Keep in mind that adequate fluid and carbohydrate intake will be critical for optimal performance on race day; however, going overboard with fluids or carbohydrates can lead to hyponatremia or a bloated, sluggish feeling on race day. Be cognizant but not excessive with your intake.

What Should You Consider the Day Before Your Race?

Be sure to do the following the day before you race:

- *Run/walk easy or take the day off.* You have two options for pre-race workouts based on how you feel:

  1. Run/walk easy for 15 minutes or around one to two miles, stretch, release nervous energy, relax, and obtain a good night's sleep.

  2. Take the day off completely and just stretch to conserve energy.

  Either option is appropriate; you decide which option will be the best.

- *Avoid foods that take longer to digest.* Do not eat fried, fatty foods or rich desserts the day before your race. These foods will sit heavy in your stomach and can make you feel sluggish or have diarrhea on race day—neither are good outcomes!

- *Don't experiment!* Now is not the time to experiment with foods, beverages, or clothing. It is important to eat the familiar foods that you have been consuming throughout your training. Choose race day clothing that you are confident will be comfortable for the duration of the race. Do not purchase a new outfit and expect to wear it "fresh" for the race—you will pay in blisters and chafing. Experimentation with different foods and clothing should occur at least one month beforehand.

- *Stay well hydrated.* Consume plenty of fluids the day before the race without going overboard. Your urine should be clear or pale in color. Your trips to the restroom should be about once every two hours—if you are urinating more frequently, back off on your fluid consumption; if you are urinating less frequently or your urine is dark in color, drink a little more.

- *Go to packet pick-up.* If possible, register early and go to packet pick-up to avoid the panic and crowds the morning of the race.

What Are the Last Minute Preparations Before the Gun Goes Off?

A little planning goes a long way the night before a race. If you prepare in advance, you will avoid the last minute panic many first-timers experience. Before you go to bed on the eve of your race, consider the following tips:

- *Set two alarms.* This event is too important to let a snooze button or alarm malfunction prevent you from achieving your goal. Put one alarm across the room so you have to physically get out of bed to turn it off. Set both alarms for a time that will allow you to dress, eat, travel, and get to the start line early.

- *Know the forecast.* For comfort and safety, you must dress appropriately before, during, and after the race. In the spring and fall, it might be crisp in the morning and a warm-up suit would be appropriate to wear before the race. Based on the length of your race, the weather may actually change while you are on the course. Therefore, you must be clothed properly to withstand changes in the air temperature and humidity levels. If it is threatening rain before, during, or after the race, you will want to pack rain gear and dry clothes for after the race.

- *Be sure to have the entry form for race day information and directions to the race.* Either online or on paper, the race entry form is typically packed with all the information you need to know for race day, including where to park and the location of the start line and restrooms.

- *Take along snacks such as fruit, bagels, granola bars, and water.* It is always a good idea to pack foods and beverages in your race morning sack. In rare occasions, races have been delayed for weather, traffic, or other unexpected reasons. By having a little snack with you, you will ensure you continue to stay well fueled until the race start. After the race, you will be thankful to have a couple of snacks in your bag to munch on before you can get home and have a well-balanced meal. Quick snacks immediately following a race also help your body expedite the recovery process.

What Should You Do to Prepare in the Hours Immediately Prior to the Race?

The necessary preparations in the hours leading up to the race can be summarized in three words—*time, familiar,* and *relax.* As mentioned several times in this chapter, allow yourself plenty of extra time to get to the race for parking, packet pick-up, restroom stops, warming up, and any unforeseen problems. If you do not give yourself enough time, the next two race morning guidelines—familiar and relax—will not happen.

Included in your race morning schedule is time for stretching and warming up. Five to ten minutes of easy walking or jogging followed by 5–10 minutes of stretching will allow your muscles to be primed and ready for the gun to go off and the race to begin. A good indication that you are warmed up properly and sufficiently is to notice that you have just broken a sweat. Do not push yourself so hard that you are fatigued before the race; get your heart rate up just enough to loosen up the muscles and joints in preparation of a 3.1, 6.2, or 13.1 mile journey. By planning ahead and scheduling time to warm-up and stretch, you can also relax (the third guideline) before heading to the starting line.

Another common race day question is, "Should I eat anything on race morning, and if I should, then what is best to eat?" This is where the familiar component is so critical. Ideally, every walker and runner would have something to eat and drink before a race to optimally fuel the body. However, not everyone has practiced with eating and drinking before exercising. The bottom line is that you should eat and drink the same thing you have had to eat and drink before your training walks and runs throughout the program. *Do not* eat or drink anything new on race day! You may not realize a product does not agree with you until halfway

before you head out the door

The following is a checklist of essential items to pack for race day:

- Vaseline or BODYGLIDE® (for under arms or thighs)
- Toilet paper (for restroom emergencies)
- Garbage bags (to wear at the start of the race if it is raining)
- Race number (you will not be allowed to begin or finish the race without an official race number!)
- Pins (to attach your race number)
- Food/gels for before, during, and after the race (to stay well-fueled and to begin the recovery process)
- Throw-away bottle filled with water or a sports beverage (to sip on before the race start)
- Money (for food, race registration, gas, shirts, and other souvenirs)
- Dry clothes (for after the race)

through your race, which could ultimately throw a wrench in your race plans. Refer to Chapter 10 for the guidelines for an optimal pre-race meal in order to concoct a meal composed of your tried-and-true foods.

The final piece of pre-race preparations is to stay relaxed. At this point, the hardest part of the event—the training—is behind you. Now it is time to enjoy the fruits of your labors. One tool to help you stay relaxed is to perform a mental rehearsal. Visualize yourself running/walking, sailing by the landmarks on the course, arriving at the finish line feeling strong, and smiling knowing you have successfully accomplished your goal. Some people like to review their anticipated *splits*—the expected times for major landmarks (that is, every mile, every 5K, and so on) along the course. Mentally review your splits only if it will not increase your anxiety level about achieving the splits. Stay positive and get fired up!

What Should You Do to Prepare in the Minutes Immediately Prior to the Race?

Ten to twenty minutes before the race, head to the start line. Do not wait until the last minute to get to the start line—give yourself some time to find out exactly where you need to go. Many races, especially the larger events, will have you line up according to your race number or your bib color in specified corrals. However, smaller races are set up on a first come, first serve basis allowing you to line up as you please. The general start line etiquette, for races with no corralling system, is to line up according to your anticipated pace with faster runners in the front and slower walkers in the back.

Regardless of the start line set-up, you need to anticipate the shoving and "dog-eat-dog" attitude that is common at the beginning of road races. It will be crowded; expect some gentle pushing or elbowing as people enter onto the course. In response to this scenario, prepare to stay calm, watch your footing, and do your best to walk/run a straight line allowing others to move around you freely.

As you did in the hours leading up to the race, relax and take some deep breaths—there is nothing more you can do, the preparation is over. Now let the hard work pay off!

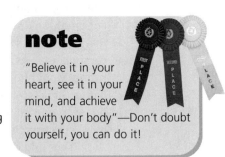

note

"Believe it in your heart, see it in your mind, and achieve it with your body"—Don't doubt yourself, you can do it!

The Gun Has Gone Off—Now What?

The race has begun and you are one step closer to achieving your goal. However, the race is not a mindless event—there are still things to think about in order to ensure you arrive successfully at the finish line. This section will provide race tips to help you deal with setting your pace, the weather conditions, course considerations, body-talk, mental chatter, and finally, the finish line.

What Do You Need to Know About Setting the Pace?

For many first-timers, when the gun goes off the natural instinct is to start off in an all-out sprint. *Resist this temptation!* The worst thing you can do is to start off too quickly, which invariably will lead to a dramatic slowing of your pace later in the race. Instead, start slow and conserve your energy, erring on the conservative side of your pace.

Many races will give you a chip to attach onto your shoelaces. This device is activated as you pass over the start line and deactivates as you cross the finish line, giving you a precise measurement of the time it took you to complete the designated course. In the old days, your official race results were based on the elapsed time from the moment the gun went off to when you crossed the finish line. In small races, this procedure may not cause any problems because all participants will cross the start line within seconds. However, some races are currently accepting 30,000 or more participants, which means it could take 5–20 minutes to even *get* to the start line! The chip alleviates the problem of having a "pre-start line" time added to your race results, providing more accurate results and allowing you to relax and not rush to the start line. If you are entered into a race that does not use the chip, anticipate the dog-eat-dog mentality to be accentuated.

tip

After the gun goes off, run/walk defensively. Watch for runners/walkers cutting in front of you, falling down or tripping, and slowing down the pace abruptly, particularly at the first few turns.

Often racers will consider going out at a faster pace than planned to give them a time cushion in order to meet their goal. Do not be tempted to make this "time in the bank" gamble. If you go out too fast in the first one or two miles you can lose more than that at the end of the race. For example, let's say your planned 10K pace is 9 minutes/mile. If you try to "bank" some time by starting off at 8:30 minute/mile pace, you could end up at a 9:30–10+ minute/mile pace by mile 4 or 5. A general rule is that for every second/mile you go out too fast in the first half of the race, you may slow by 2–10 seconds/mile in the last half of the race. In extreme cases, you could *hit the wall;* a phrase that describes the feeling of completely running out of gas, causing you to slow down or even stop. Start conservatively. You can always pick up the pace to walk/run faster as the race progresses, if you are feeling good.

What happens if you didn't intend to implement the "time in the bank" theory but at mile one you are 15–30 seconds faster than your planned race pace? Don't worry; your race is not over. If you go out too fast, slow your pace to 5–10 seconds/mile below your planned pace for one or two miles until you begin to recover, and then resume your normal pace. When you have returned to your planned pace, attempt to run/walk an even pace as much as possible for the remainder of the race. Deviations in pace, such as constantly speeding up and slowing down, are an inefficient use of a limited supply of energy.

What Do You Need to Know About the Weather Conditions?

Do not race in a vacuum; you must adapt your race plans to the weather conditions (heat and wind) of the day. On hot days, slow your pace, stay well hydrated, and listen to your body (see Table 12.1). Watch for shade (trees, buildings, and so on) on the course to cool you down. Often spectators will be on the course with sprinklers and hoses. While the thought of running through cold water may sound refreshing, think twice before getting wet. If you get soaked by sprinkles or hoses, you will have to carry a lot of extra weight in your water-soaked clothes and shoes and possibly develop blisters. In general, drinking water versus dancing through water will keep you cool and comfortable on the course.

caution

Above 85 degrees, there is an increased risk for heat related illness—run/walk easy, stay well-hydrated, monitor your body, and toss your preconceived time goals out the window!

Table 12.1 Adjusting Your Race Pace in the Heat

Estimated Temperature at Finish	Slower than Goal Pace	10 Min/Mile Pace Becomes
55–60 degrees	1%	10:05
60–65 degrees	3%	10:15
65–70 degrees	5%	10:25
70–75 degrees	7%	10:35
75–80 degrees	12%	10:58
80–85 degrees	20%	11:35

In windy conditions, lean slightly forward, use your arms, do not bounce (stay close to the ground), and watch for wind-blockers (such as buildings or other racers). Consider "drafting," which involves running or walking 2–6 feet behind other racers to block the wind. Drafting can save 1%–2% of your energy, which can become significant in a long race such as the half-marathon!

What Do You Need to Know About the Course?

Exploring the race course in the days leading up to the race will give you a good idea of what to expect on race day. In addition to your visual memory of the course, there are a few other tips that will help you move with ease and efficiency from start line to finish line:

- Run/walk the tangents (the shortest distance between two points) so you don't waste any energy going longer than necessary.

- For uphills, walk/run the same number of strides per minute but shorten your strides, lift your knees, use your arms, and lean slightly forward.

- For downhills, run/walk the same number of strides per minutes but lengthen your strides, relax, and "roll," while resisting the temptation to pick up the pace.

- Stay on the flat part of the course (crown or gutter); walking/running on uneven pavement will cause hip, knee, or ankle pain over time.

- Be alert for potholes, grates, traffic, cones, and other debris or obstacles on the course—especially if you are drafting!

- When taking fluids, watch for wet spots, cups, and racers going to and from water stations; to avoid the traffic and congestion, go to the last table and slow down or walk to take in fluids.

- Know where the portable toilets and medical tents are located, just in case you need them.

tip

When taking fluids on the course, pick up a cup and then scrunch the cup on two sides to form a spout to pour the fluids more effectively into your mouth. This method will dramatically increase the amount of fluid ingested and greatly reduce the amount of water or sports drinks that ends up on your race outfit!

What Do You Need to Know About Your "Body Talk"?

During the race, listen to your body. Pay attention to your muscles, breathing, degree of perspiration, and energy level and then adjust your pace accordingly. It is important to emphasize how your body feels versus the split times on your watch in order to prevent injuries. If you experience unusual or persistent pain or symptoms (such as gastrointestinal problems, severe cramps, lightheadedness, and so on) seek medical assistance. Do not try to tough it out. Some physical distractions such as minor muscle soreness and slight fatigue are common. The solutions to these minor physical distractions include slowing your pace and setting short-term goals (such as going from one mile marker or water station to the next). One of the most frequently experienced physical distractions is the side stitch. While the causes and cures are not proven, one theory to alleviate side stitches is to exhale forcefully (grunt!) when you land with the foot opposite the stitch side. This remedy may not work every time, but it won't hurt to try.

What Do You Need to Know About Your Mental Chatter?

The mind is a powerful thing. If your attitude and drive begin to droop, your performance will suffer. To avoid breaking down mentally during your race, consider the following ways to positively alter your mental chatter:

- *Choose positive over negative self-talk.* For example, tell yourself, "I can," "I feel good," "Seven down and six to go," or "Piece of cake!," to keep you moving strong toward the finish line.

- *Associating versus disassociating.* Either technique can work based on your personal preferences and outlook on life. Associating means that you strengthen your focus by thinking about what you are doing, watching the clock, listening to your body, and being aware of those around you. Disassociating means that you start thinking about work, family, your next vacation, or how you will celebrate when the race is over to keep your mind occupied and your body moving forward.

  tip

  "Race to the beat of your own drummer"—know your race plan and stick to it!

- *Break the race up into segments.* It can be less overwhelming to think of your race in smaller chunks such as: 3×1 mile + 0.1 miles for a 5K race; $2 \times 5K$ for a 10K race; and $4 \times 5Ks + 1.1$ or $2 \times 10Ks + 0.7$ for a half-marathon.

■ *Set your sights on the runner/walker in front of you.* Let other racers "pull you" through while being careful not to deviate too much from your original plan.

■ *Station friends, family, and co-workers at key locations.* Position your support crew on the course in challenging locations such as the hills or the last few miles. Have them play the "Rocky" theme song as you pass by.

■ *Consistent pacing.* Watch out for passing games played by walkers or runners who are inefficient, making dramatic increases and decreases in their pace. Instead, work together to help one another through the race.

What Do You Need to Know About the Finish Line?

When the race is over, stop your watch, look at the clock, and keep moving through the chute. Once you are through the chute, resist the temptation to sit down. Instead, keep moving to decrease muscle soreness later in the day due to lactic acid build-up. Pre-arrange an area to meet friends and family. Together you can cool down and stretch. It is also important to eat and drink immediately, however slowly, after the finish to begin the repair and replenishment process. Have a snack at the finish line and then within two hours, eat a well-balanced meal containing carbohydrates, protein, and fluids.

What Is the Best Way to Recover from the Race?

The recovery process in the hours and days after the race can be greatly affected by your actions. Active rest and nutrition are the key concepts. Later that day, after the race, go for a walk or try window shopping—something slow and easy, but active to flush out your muscles. Stretch lightly before going to bed and when you wake up the next morning to loosen up your muscles and joints. The day after the race, you can try to jog or walk easy but do not go further than about 15 minutes or around one or two miles. Your second option is to continue to rest, but make it an active rest as you did the day before.

In terms of nutrition, hydration and balanced meals should be your focus. Continue to rehydrate while being careful not to overhydrate. Remember, your urine should be pale in color with bathroom breaks once every two to three hours. If your urge to urinate is more frequent, back off your fluid consumption slightly. Your meals should incorporate a carbohydrate and protein source to ensure the replenishment of your glycogen stores and the repair of muscles.

THE ABSOLUTE MINIMUM

- A week before the race, drive the course and check out places to park for race morning.

- Two days before the race, get a good night's sleep and start loading up on fluids and carbohydrates.

- The day before the race, either run/walk easy or take the day off. Stay well hydrated, eat only familiar foods, and go to packet pick-up (if possible).

- Pack a bag of your essential items for race day the night before the race.

- Stay relaxed and enjoy the race experience.

- Be a defensive walker/runner and aim to keep an even pace throughout the race.

- Use active rest and proper nutrition to help you recover quickly and completely.

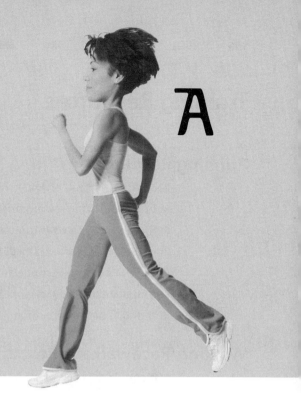

ADDITIONAL RESOURCES AND LOGS

Training Resources

The following sections provide training resources for runners and walkers.

Running Resources

Road Runners Club of America, www.rrca.org

Running Online, www.runningonline.com

Running Network, www.runningnetwork.com

Run the Planet, www.runtheplanet.com

Runner's World, www.runnersworld.com

Running Magazine, www.splittimes.com

Running Times, www.runningtimes.com

Walking/Racewalking Resources

National Masters News, www.nationalmastersnews.com

Racewalk, www.racewalk.com

Walking Magazine, www.walkingmag.com

World Wide Walkers, www.worldwidewalkers.net

Walking and Running Resources

Active Network, www.active.com

American Running and Fitness Association, www.americanrunning.org

Nationwide events, www.coolrunning.com

Run Walk Jog, www.runwalkjog.com

USA Track & Field, www.usatf.org

Fundraisers for Health

American Heart Walk, www.amhrt.org

America's Walk for Diabetes, http://walk.diabetes.org

Koman Breast Cancer Foundation, www.raceforthecure.com

Leukemia & Lymphoma Society, www.teamintraining.org

Relay for Life, www.cancerrelay.com

Schoolwalk for Diabetes, www.diabetes.org/schoolwalk

Sports Nutrition Resources

The following sections provide sports nutrition resources for runners and walkers.

Newsletters

Gatorade Sports Sciences Exchange. 617 W. Main Street, Barrington, IL 60604-9005. A monthly newsletter that reviews the current research on sports nutrition topics. www.gssiweb.com

Running and Fit News. 4405 East West Highway, Bethesda, MD 20814. American Running and Fitness Association. www.americanrunning.org

SCAN's Pulse. American Dietetic Association, P.O. Box 60820, Colorado Springs, CO 80960. Newsletter of the Sports, Cardiovascular & Wellness Nutritionists. www.scandpg.org

Professional Organizations

American Dietetic Association. 120 S. Riverside Plaza, Suite 2000, Chicago, IL 60606-6995. Phone: 1-800-877-1600, www.eatright.org

American College of Sports Medicine. 401 West Michigan, Indianapolis, IN 46202. Phone: 317-637-9200, www.acsm.org

American Running and Fitness Association. 4405 East West Highway, Suite 405, Bethesda, MD 20814. Phone: 301-913-9517, www.americanrunning.org

Books

Clark, N. (2003). *Nancy Clark's Sports Nutrition Guidebook,* 3rd Edition.

Clark, N. (1994). *The NYC Marathon Cookbook: A Nutrition Guide for Runners.*

Colberg, S. (2000). *The Diabetic Athlete.*

Coleman, E. (1988). *Eating for Endurance.*

Dorfman, L. (2000). *The Vegetarian Sports Nutrition Guidebook.*

Duyff, R. (2002). *The American Dietetic Association's Complete Food & Nutrition Guide,* 2nd Edition.

Gordon, N. (1993). *Diabetes: Your Complete Exercise Guide.*

Noakes, T. (2003). *The Lore of Running,* 4th Edition.

Websites

American College of Sports Medicine, www.acsm.org

American Dietetic Association, www.eatright.org

American Running and Fitness, www.americanrunning.org

Department of Health and Human Services, www.dhhs.gov

Food and Nutrition Information Center, www.nal.usda.gov/fnic/

Gatorade Sports Science Institute, www.gssiweb.com

Human Kinetics, www.humankinetics.com

National Council Against Health Fraud (NCAHF), www.ncahf.org

National Health Information Center, www.health.gov/nhic/

National Institutes of Health, www.nih.gov

National Strength and Conditioning, www.nsca.org

Sports, Cardiovascular & Wellness Nutritionists, www.scandpg.org

Sports Medicine Magazine, www.physsportsmed.com

Sports Nutrition: Ask the Dietitian, www.dietitian.com/sportnut.html

Training and Nutrition Logs

Use these logs to keep track of your 5K, 10K, half-marathon, and strength-training progress and to chart your nutritional intake as you prepare for race day. Printable PDF versions of each of these logs are available for download from this book's web page at http://www.quepublishing.com/. Type this book's ISBN (0789733145) into the Search field to go to this book's web page, you will find printable PDF versions of all three of these logs available for download.

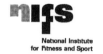

Strength Training Log

NAME		DATE __/__/__	DATE __/__/__	DATE __/__/__	DATE __/__/__	DATE __/__/__	DATE __/__/__
EXERCISE		WT/REPS	WT/REPS	WT/REPS	WT/REPS	WT/REPS	WT/REPS
UPPER BODY	1 2 3 4						
	1 2 3 4						
	1 2 3 4						
	1 2 3 4						
LOWER BODY	1 2 3 4						
	1 2 3 4						
	1 2 3 4						
	1 2 3 4						
ABDOMINALS / BACK	1 2 3 4						
	1 2 3 4						
	1 2 3 4						
	1 2 3 4						

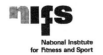

National Institute
for Fitness and Sport

Strength Training Log

NAME			DATE __/__/__	DATE __/__/__	DATE __/__/__	DATE __/__/__	DATE __/__/__	DATE __/__/__
EXERCISE			WT/REPS	WT/REPS	WT/REPS	WT/REPS	WT/REPS	WT/REPS
UPPER BODY		1 2 3 4						
		1 2 3 4						
		1 2 3 4						
		1 2 3 4						
LOWER BODY		1 2 3 4						
		1 2 3 4						
		1 2 3 4						
		1 2 3 4						
ABDOMINALS / BACK		1 2 3 4						
		1 2 3 4						
		1 2 3 4						
		1 2 3 4						

Training Log

MONDAY				
DATE	DURATION	DISTANCE	HEART RATE	TEMP
COMMENTS (i.e. type of exercise; pace):				

TUESDAY				
DATE	DURATION	DISTANCE	HEART RATE	TEMP
COMMENTS (i.e. type of exercise; pace):				

WEDNESDAY				
DATE	DURATION	DISTANCE	HEART RATE	TEMP
COMMENTS (i.e. type of exercise; pace):				

THURSDAY				
DATE	DURATION	DISTANCE	HEART RATE	TEMP
COMMENTS (i.e. type of exercise; pace):				

FRIDAY				
DATE	DURATION	DISTANCE	HEART RATE	TEMP
COMMENTS (i.e. type of exercise; pace):				

SATURDAY				
DATE	DURATION	DISTANCE	HEART RATE	TEMP
COMMENTS (i.e. type of exercise; pace):				

SUNDAY				
DATE	DURATION	DISTANCE	HEART RATE	TEMP
COMMENTS (i.e. type of exercise; pace):				

SUMMARY		
WEEK'S TOTAL	MONTH'S TOTAL	YEAR'S TOTAL
LONGEST RUN-WALK	SHORTEST RUN-WALK	AVERAGE RUN-WALK

Training Log

MONDAY				
DATE	**DURATION**	**DISTANCE**	**HEART RATE**	**TEMP**
COMMENTS (i.e. type of exercise; pace):				

TUESDAY				
DATE	**DURATION**	**DISTANCE**	**HEART RATE**	**TEMP**
COMMENTS (i.e. type of exercise; pace):				

WEDNESDAY				
DATE	**DURATION**	**DISTANCE**	**HEART RATE**	**TEMP**
COMMENTS (i.e. type of exercise; pace):				

THURSDAY				
DATE	**DURATION**	**DISTANCE**	**HEART RATE**	**TEMP**
COMMENTS (i.e. type of exercise; pace):				

FRIDAY				
DATE	DURATION	DISTANCE	HEART RATE	TEMP
COMMENTS (i.e. type of exercise; pace):				

SATURDAY				
DATE	DURATION	DISTANCE	HEART RATE	TEMP
COMMENTS (i.e. type of exercise; pace):				

SUNDAY				
DATE	DURATION	DISTANCE	HEART RATE	TEMP
COMMENTS (i.e. type of exercise; pace):				

SUMMARY		
WEEK'S TOTAL	MONTH'S TOTAL	YEAR'S TOTAL
LONGEST RUN-WALK	SHORTEST RUN-WALK	AVERAGE RUN-WALK

The National Institute for Fitness and Sport - Weekly Food Record

Goals for the week: _____

	BREAKFAST	LUNCH	DINNER	SNACKS
SAMPLE	• 2 slices of whole wheat toast (2 grains) • 1 t margarine (1 fat) • banana (1 fruit) • 6 oz. orange juice (1 fruit)	• Chicken Caesar Salad – 2 oz. grilled chicken (1 meat) – 2 cups mixed greens (2 veg.) – 1 tb. caesar dressing (1 fat) • 2 breadsticks (2 grains) • 1 cup yogurt (1 milk)	• 3 oz. grilled chicken (1 meat) • 1/2 cup cooked brown rice (1 grain) • 1 t margarine (1 fat) • 1/2 cup cooked broccoli (1 veg.) • 8 oz. skim milk (1 milk)	• 1 oz. mini pretzels (1 grain) • 2 chocolate chip cookies (2 fat) • 6 oz. grape fruit juice (1 fruit)
MONDAY				
TUESDAY				
WEDNESDAY				

SAMPLE — Grain- Vegetable- [SERVINGS] Meat- Sugar- -Fat -Milk -Fruit

MONDAY — Grain- Vegetable- [SERVINGS] Meat- Sugar- -Fat -Milk -Fruit

TUESDAY — Grain- Vegetable- [SERVINGS] Meat- Sugar- -Fat -Milk -Fruit

WEDNESDAY — Grain- Vegetable- [SERVINGS] Meat- Sugar- -Fat -Milk -Fruit

The National Institute for Fitness and Sport - Weekly Food Record

Goals for the week: _____

	BREAKFAST	LUNCH	DINNER	SNACKS
THURSDAY Sugar- Meat- -Fat -Milk SERVINGS Vegetable- -Fruit Grain-				
FRIDAY Sugar- Meat- -Fat -Milk SERVINGS Vegetable- -Fruit Grain-				
SATURDAY Sugar- Meat- -Fat -Milk SERVINGS Vegetable- -Fruit Grain-				
SUNDAY Sugar- Meat- -Fat -Milk SERVINGS Vegetable- -Fruit Grain-				

The National Institute for Fitness and Sport - Weekly Food Record

Goals for the week:

	BREAKFAST	LUNCH	DINNER	SNACKS

SAMPLE
 	
Grain-
Vegetable-
SERVINGS
Sugar-
Meat-
 	
-Fat
-Milk
-Fruit
	• 2 slices of whole wheat toast (2 grains)
	• 1 t margarine (1 fat)
	• banana (1 fruit)
	• 6 oz. orange juice (1 fruit)
		• Chicken Caesar Salad
		  – 2 oz. grilled chicken (1 meat)
		  – 2 cups mixed greens (2 veg.)
		  – 1 tb. caesar dressing (1 fat)
		• 2 breadsticks (2 grains)
		• 1 cup yogurt (1 milk)
			• 3 oz. grilled chicken (1 meat)
			• 1/2 cup cooked brown rice (1 grain)
			• 1 t margarine (1 fat)
			• 1/2 cup cooked broccoli (1 veg.)
			• 8 oz. skim milk (1 milk)
				• 1 oz. mini pretzels (1 grain)
				• 2 chocolate chip cookies (2 fat)
				• 6 oz. grape fruit juice (1 fruit)

MONDAY Grain- Vegetable- **SERVINGS** Sugar- Meat- -Fat -Milk -Fruit				
TUESDAY Grain- Vegetable- **SERVINGS** Sugar- Meat- -Fat -Milk -Fruit				
WEDNESDAY Grain- Vegetable- **SERVINGS** Sugar- Meat- -Fat -Milk -Fruit				

The National Institute for Fitness and Sport - Weekly Food Record

Goals for the week: _____

	BREAKFAST	LUNCH	DINNER	SNACKS
THURSDAY SERVINGS Grain- Vegetable- Meat- Sugar- -Fat -Milk -Fruit				
FRIDAY SERVINGS Grain- Vegetable- Meat- Sugar- -Fat -Milk -Fruit				
SATURDAY SERVINGS Grain- Vegetable- Meat- Sugar- -Fat -Milk -Fruit				
SUNDAY SERVINGS Grain- Vegetable- Meat- Sugar- -Fat -Milk -Fruit				

Index

How can we make this index more useful? Email us at indexes@quepublishing.com

How can we make this index more useful? Email us at indexes@quepublishing.com

How can we make this index more useful? Email us at indexes@quepublishing.com

I - J - K

L

N

How can we make this index more useful? Email us at indexes@quepublishing.com

orthopedic limitations, injury prevention, 59

paces

setting during races, 179-180

weather conditions, 180-181

poor program design, injury prevention, 60

post-workout activities

electrolyte replacement, 162

recommended carbohydrate intake, 161

recommended fluids, 161

recommended foods, 160

recommended protein intake, 161-162

pre-race meals

digestion times, 150-151

healthy snack/meal ideas, 151

reasons for, 148

recommended foods, 149

pre-race strategies

day prior checklist, 175-176

immediate preparations checklist, 177-178

last minute checklist, 176-178

week prior checklist, 174

progression of intensity, injury prevention, 55

proper form, 76

arm swing, 78

high stride rate, 77

maximized breathing, 78-79

overstriding prevention, 76-77

posture, 78

stride length optimization, 76

vertical oscillation, 78

race courses

strategies, 181

water stations, 181

race day, essentials checklist, 177

races

mental chatter, countering, 182-183

monitoring body for ailments, 182

recovery process, 183

reflective gear

Adidas Adistar Rain Jacket, 50

Nathan & Co. Reflective Safety Vest, 50

New Balance Tepid Training Vest, 50

Petzl Tikka Plus Headlamp, 50

Road ID BrightGear, 50

Road ID Shoe ID, 50

RSS Reflective Kit, 50

Sugoi Microfine Reflective Cap, 50

returning from prior injury, 60

safety devices, injury prevention, 58-59

safety hints, 52

shoe selection, injury prevention, 57-58

side stitches, treating, 182

speed work, injury prevention, 55-56

stretching, injury prevention, 56

warm-ups, importance of, 84

Running and Fit newsletter, 187

***Running Magazine* website, 186**

Running Network website, 186

Running Online website, 186

running shoes

fitting guidelines, 40

versus walking shoes, 41

running sites

National Masters News, 186

Road Runners Club of America, 186

Run the Planet, 186

Runner's World, 186

Running Magazine, 186

Running Network, 186

Running Online, 186

Running Times, 186

Running Times website, 186

How can we make this index more useful? Email us at indexes@quepublishing.com

T

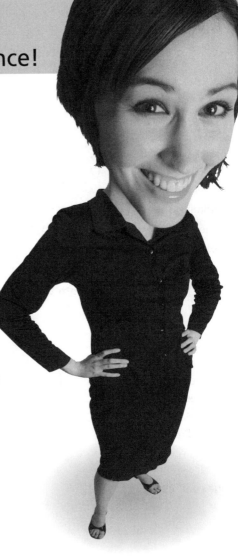
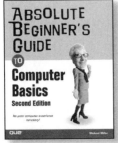
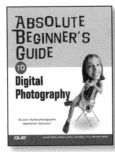
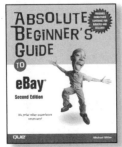
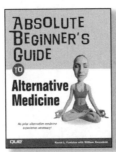
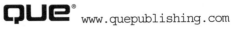